A Concise Guide to Observational Studies in Healthcare

T0176288

A Concise Guide to Observational Studies in Healthcare

Allan Hackshaw

University College London
London
UK

WILEY Blackwell   BMJ|Books

Library of Congress Cataloging-in-Publication Data
Hackshaw, Allan K., author.
  A concise guide to observational studies in healthcare / Allan Hackshaw.
    p. ; cm.
  Includes bibliographical references and index.
  ISBN 978-0-470-65867-3 (pbk.)
  I. Title.
  [DNLM: 1. Observational Study as Topic–methods–Handbooks. 2. Outcome and Process
Assessment (Health Care)–Handbooks. 3. Epidemiologic Research Design–Handbooks. W 49]
  R852
  610.72–dc23
                                        2014018407
A catalogue record for this book is available from the British Library.

Contents

Foreword

Epidemiology is at the heart of medicine. Without knowledge of the epidemiology of disease and its methods of study, it can be impossible to interpret the results of observational studies. Epidemiology has an important role to play in determining causes of disease and in the interpretation of clinical tests since this depends on knowledge of the prevalence of the diseases for which such tests are done. Observational studies are the mainstay of epidemiology. Correctly interpreted, observational studies transform the unstructured natural variation of diseases and the exposures that cause them into intelligible insights that can be used to improve health and well-being. *A Concise Guide to Observational Studies in Healthcare* demonstrates how this is done and includes many practical examples.

It is easy to complicate epidemiology with mathematical formulae and specialist jargons that are difficult to understand. What are the differences between relative risk, odds ratio and hazard ratio? What is the difference between bias and confounding? How should a meta-analysis be presented and interpreted? Why are the terms detection rate and false positive rate better than sensitivity and specificity? What is the difference between a standard deviation and a standard error? Hackshaw carefully explains all these and more with elegance. The book succeeds in pulling together the essence of how observational studies can be used and interpreted in medical practice.

Hackshaw simplifies the principles and methods of the subject, covering a wide range of topics in a book short enough to be read over a weekend and one that will undoubtedly inspire readers to delve further into the subject.

A Concise Guide to Observational Studies in Healthcare is a useful companion to Hackshaw's 2009 book on clinical trials. As with his previous book, this one is aimed at the general, medical and scientific reader, providing an introduction to the subject without requiring detailed specialist knowledge, an objective the author has accomplished with skill and rigour.

Professor Sir Nicholas Wald, FRS, FRCP
Wolfson Institute of Preventive Medicine
Barts and The London School of Medicine and Dentistry

Preface

Research studies are required for developing effective public health policies and clinical practice. Observational studies are perhaps the most common type of research, and they are essential for describing the characteristics of a group of people or finding ways to understand, detect, prevent or treat disease, or avert early death.

The purpose of the book is to provide researchers and health professionals with a focussed and simplified account of the main features of observational studies. It is important to first understand the key concepts. Specifics about the calculations involved in analyses should come after and are covered in other textbooks. The book is aimed at those who conduct their own studies or participate in studies coordinated by others, or to help review a published report. No prior knowledge of design, analysis or conduct is required. Examples are based on clinical features of people, biomarkers, lifestyle habits and environmental exposures, and evaluating quality of care.

This book is a companion to the book *A Concise Guide to Clinical Trials* (Hackshaw A, BMJ Books/Wiley-Blackwell). An overview of the key design and analytical features are provided in Chapters 1–4; then each study type is discussed using published studies (Chapters 5–8), showing how they were conducted and interpreted. Chapter 9 introduces prognostic markers, a topic which is often misunderstood, while Chapter 10 covers systematic reviews and how to deal with inconsistent results. Chapter 11 summarises how to conduct and publish an observational study.

One of the important goals of the book is to show that study features such as the design of questionnaires and interpreting results are common to most study types, so these topics are repeated throughout the chapters. By having many examples, the reader can see how a variety of study designs and outcomes can be interpreted in a similar way, which will help to reinforce key aspects.

The content is based on over 23 years of experience teaching evidence-based medicine to undergraduates, postgraduates, and health professionals; writing over 130 published articles in books and medical journals; and designing, setting up and analysing research studies for a variety of disorders. This background has provided the experience to determine what researchers need to know and how to present the relevant ideas.

I am most grateful to Jan Mackie, whose thorough editing of the book was invaluable. Final thanks to Harald Bauer.

Professor Allan Hackshaw
Deputy Director Cancer Research UK & UCL Cancer Trials Centre
University College London

CHAPTER 1

Fundamental concepts

This chapter provides a summary background to observational studies, their main purposes, the common types of designs, and some key design features. Further details on design and analysis are illustrated using examples in later chapters, and from other textbooks [1–3].

1.1 Observational studies: purpose

Two distinct study designs are used in medical research: **observational** and **experimental**. Experimental studies, commonly called clinical trials, are specifically designed to intervene in some aspect of how the study participants live their life or how they are treated in order to evaluate a health-related outcome. A key feature of a clinical trial is that some or all participants receive an intervention that they would not normally be given. Observational studies, as the term implies, are not intentionally meant to intervene in the way individuals live or behave or how they are treated.[#] Participants are free to choose their lifestyle habits and, with their physician, decide which interventions they receive when considering preventing or treating a disorder. Box 1.1 shows the most common purposes of observational studies.

1.2 Specifying a clear research question: exposures and outcomes

The **research question(s)**, which can also be referred to as **objectives**, **purpose**, **aims**, or **hypotheses**, should be clear, easy to read, and written in non-technical language where possible. They are usually developed to address a research issue that has not been examined before, to corroborate or refute previous evidence, or to examine a topic on which prior evidence has had shortcomings or been scientifically flawed.

[#]Though in reality, just by being in a study could alter someone's behaviour or lifestyle habits.

A Concise Guide to Observational Studies in Healthcare, First Edition. Allan Hackshaw.
© 2015 John Wiley & Sons, Ltd. Published 2015 by John Wiley & Sons, Ltd.

Box 1.1 Common purposes of observational studies

• Examine the opinions of a single group of people on a health-related topic(s)
• Describe the health-related characteristics (e.g. demographics, lifestyle habits, genes, biological measurement, or imaging marker) of a single group of people
• Estimate the occurrence of a disorder at a given time, or trends over time
• Examine features of a disorder (e.g. how it affects patient's lives, how they are managed/treated, and short- or long-term consequences)
• Find associations between the health-related characteristics among a single group of people or across two or more groups
• Examine risk factors (including casual factors) for a disorder or early death
• Examine prognostic factors (i.e. those that can predict the occurrence of a disorder or death from the disorder)
• Evaluate a healthcare intervention for prevention or treatment

Find new scientific information
Plan the use of future resources
Change public health education, policy, or practice
Change clinical practice

Disease prevention, detection, or treatment

There is a distinction between **objectives** and **outcome measures** (or **endpoints**). An outcome measure is the specific quantitative measure used to address the objective. For example, a study objective could be 'to examine the smoking habits of adults'. Possible corresponding endpoints could be either 'the proportion of all participants who report themselves as smokers' or 'the number of cigarettes smoked per day', but they are quite different endpoints. Box 1.2 shows examples of objectives and outcome measures.

It can be easy to specify the research question or objective for studies that involve simply describing the characteristics of a single group of people (e.g. demographics, or biological or physical measurements). For example:
• What proportion of pregnant women give birth at home?
• What is the distribution of blood pressure and serum cholesterol measurements among men and women aged over 50?

Box 1.2 Examples of objectives and outcome measures (endpoints)

Objective	Outcome measure
To examine the effectiveness of statin therapy in people with no history of heart disease	Mean serum cholesterol level
To evaluate blood pressure as a risk factor for stroke	The occurrence (incidence) of stroke
To examine the smoking and alcohol drinking habits of medical students	The number of cigarettes smoked per day and the number of alcohol units consumed in a week
To determine whether there is an association between arthritis and coffee consumption	The occurrence of arthritis
To examine the association between age and blood pressure	Age and blood pressure measured on every subject

- Are patients satisfied with the quality of care received in a cancer clinic?

Clinical trials often have a single primary objective, occasionally two or three at most, each associated with an endpoint. However, there can be more flexibility on this for observational studies unless they have been designed to change a specific aspect of public health policy. Many observational studies have several objectives, some of which may only arise during the study or at the end, and they can also be exploratory.

Examining the effect of an exposure on an outcome

While some researchers seek only to describe the characteristics of a single group of people (the simplest study type), it is common to look at associations between two factors. Many research studies, both observational studies and clinical trials, are designed to:

Examine the effect of an *exposure* on an *outcome*

Box 1.3 gives examples of these. To evaluate risk factors or causes of disease or early death, an outcome measure must be compared between two groups of people:
1. Exposed group
2. Unexposed group

Box 1.3 Examples of studies examining the effect of an exposure on an outcome

	Exposure	Outcome*
Exposures (characteristics) that cannot be changed or modified	Age	Heart disease
	BRCA1/BRCA2 gene	Breast cancer
	Family history	Alzheimer's disease
	Prostate specific antigen	Prostate cancer
	Burn size after an accident	Mortality
Exposures (characteristics) that can be changed or modified	Alcohol	Arthritis (gout)
	Frequent mobile phone use	Brain cancer
	Working with asbestos	Mesothelioma
	Body weight	Diabetes
Interventions	A new diet for obese people	**Body weight**
	Epileptic drugs during pregnancy	Birth defect
	Being treated in A&E at weekends	Death within 7 days

A&E, accident and emergency department.

Body weight is highlighted to show that a factor can be either an outcome or exposure, depending on the research question:

'What is the effect of body weight on the risk of developing diabetes?'

'What is the effect of a new diet on body weight'

*The risk of developing the specified disorder, except body weight which is a continuous measurement so there is no direct concept of risk.

An exposure is often thought to be a factor that can be avoided or removed from our lives, such as a lifestyle habit or something encountered at work or in the environment, but it can be any of the following:

- Physical or clinical characteristic
- Gene or genetic mutation
- Biomarker (measured in blood, saliva, or tissue)
- Imaging marker
- Intervention for prevention or treatment

Also, a factor can be either an exposure or an outcome, depending on the research question (e.g. body weight in Box 1.3). Considering a research study in the context of examining the relationship between exposures and outcomes greatly helps to understand the design and analysis.

"Make everything else the same": natural variation, confounding, and bias

An important consideration for all observational research studies is **variability** (**natural variation**). For example, smoking is a cause of lung cancer, but why do some people who have smoked 40 cigarettes a day for most of their adult lives not develop lung cancer, while others who have never smoked do? The answer is that people **vary**. They have different body characteristics (e.g. weight and blood pressure), different genetic make-up, and different lifestyles (e.g. diet, and exercise). People react to the same exposure in different ways.

When an association (risk or causal factor)[#] is evaluated, it is essential to consider if the observed responses are consistent with natural variation or whether there really is an effect. Allowance must be made for variability in order to judge how much of the association seen at the end of a study is due to natural variation (i.e. chance) and how much is due to the effect of the risk factor of interest. The more variability there is, the harder it is to detect an association. Highly controlled studies (such as laboratory experiments or randomised clinical trials) have relatively less variation because the researchers have control over how the study subjects (biological samples, animals, or human participants) are selected, managed, and assessed.

The best way to evaluate the effect of an exposure on an outcome is to 'make everything the same', in relation to the characteristics of the two (or more) groups being compared except the factor of interest. For example, to examine whether smoking is a cause of lung cancer, the risk of lung cancer between never-smokers and current smokers must be compared; to evaluate statin therapy for treating people with ischaemic heart disease, survival times between patients who did and did not receive statins are compared. Ideally, the exposed and unexposed groups should be identical in terms of demographics, physical and biological characteristics, and lifestyle habits, so that the <u>only</u> difference between the groups is that one is exposed to the factor of interest (smokes or receives statins) and the other is not exposed. [In reality, the two groups can never be identical; there will always be some random (chance) differences between them due to natural variability.] Consequently, if a clear difference is seen in the outcome measure (lung cancer risk or survival time), it should only be due to the exposure status, and not any other factor. This is a fundamental concept in medical research, and one that allows **causal** inferences to be made more reliably. An example is shown in Box 1.4.

In a randomised clinical trial, the process of randomisation aims to 'make everything the same', except the intervention given. The researcher randomly allocates the interventions (exposures) leading to two similar groups. Any

---

[#] Presented in Chapter 2

Box 1.4 Illustration of how differences between exposed and unexposed groups influence the effect of an exposure on an outcome measure

	Exposed: smokers	Unexposed: never-smokers
	N = 2500	N = 7500
Eat lots of fruit and vegetables	25%	60%
Had heart attack	10%	5%

Interest is only in examining the effect of smoking on the risk of a heart attack. The risk is twice as high among smokers than never-smokers, so we could conclude that smoking is associated with heart disease. But it is not possible to distinguish whether this difference (effect) could be due to:
- The difference in smoking status
- The difference in diet
- A combination of the two

---

differences in the outcome measure should only be due to the intervention, which is why clinical trials (and systematic reviews of them) usually provide the best level of evidence in medical research, and a causal relationship can often be determined. Published reports of all randomised studies contain a table confirming that baseline characteristics are similar between the trial groups.

In observational studies, however, the exposure cannot be randomly allocated by the research team. The researchers can only <u>observe</u>, not intervene, and it is likely for several differences to exist between the groups to be compared. The more differences there are, the more difficult it will be to conclude a causal link. The two main sources of these differences are **confounding** and **bias**. Confounding and bias might still be present to some small extent in a randomised clinical trial, but the purpose of randomisation is to minimise their effect.

Confounding and bias can each distort the results and therefore the conclusions (Box 1.5).

Some researchers consider confounding as a type of bias, because both have similar effects on the results. However, a key difference is that it is usually possible to measure confounding factors and therefore allow for them in the statistical analysis, but a factor associated with bias is often difficult or impossible to measure, and therefore it cannot be adjusted for in the same way as confounding. Confounding and bias could work together, or in opposite directions. It may not be possible to separate their effects reliably.

Researchers try to remove or minimise the effect of bias at the design stage or when conducting the study. The effect of some confounding factors can also be minimised at this stage (**matched case–control studies**, see Chapter 6, page 114).

Box 1.5 Confounding and bias

• **Confounding** represents the natural relationships between physical and biochemical characteristics, genetic make-up, and lifestyle and habits, which may affect how an individual responds to an exposure.
• It cannot be removed from a research study, but known confounding factors can be allowed for in a statistical analysis if they have been measured, or at the design stage (matched case–control studies).

• **Bias** is usually a design feature of a study that affects how participants are selected, treated, managed, or assessed.
• It often arises through the actions of the study participants and/or the research team.
• The effect of bias could be minimised or prevented by careful study design and conduct, but human nature makes this difficult.
• It is difficult, sometimes impossible, to allow for bias in a statistical analysis because it cannot be measured reliably.

The confounding and bias factors themselves are relatively unimportant. What matters more is whether they greatly influence the study results:
• Make an effect appear spuriously, when in reality there is no association
• Overestimate the magnitude of an effect
• Underestimate the magnitude of an effect
• Hide a real effect

Confounding

A confounding factor is often another type of exposure, and to affect the study results, it must be associated with both the exposure and outcome of interest (Figure 1.1). The factor could be more common in either the exposed or unexposed groups.

Figure 1.2 shows a hypothetical example of how confounding can distort the results of a study. The primary interest is in whether smoking is associated with death from liver cirrhosis. In Figure 1.2a, if the death rates are simply compared between smokers and non-smokers, they appear to be higher among smokers (15 vs. 9 per 1000). It could be concluded that smokers have a higher risk, and this could be used as supporting evidence that smoking is a risk factor for cirrhosis. However, from Figure 1.2a, it is clear that smokers are more likely to be alcohol drinkers (66 vs. 34%), and it is already known that alcohol increases the risk of liver cirrhosis. Because the exposed (current smokers) and unexposed (never-smokers) groups have different alcohol consumption habits, they are not 'the same', and the difference in death rates could be due to smoking status, the difference in alcohol consumption, or a combination of the two.

Because drinking status has been measured for all participants, it is perhaps intuitive that to remove its confounding effect, the association between smoking and cirrhosis deaths can be examined *separately* for drinkers and non-drinkers.

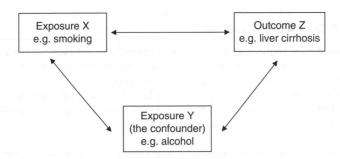

A confounder Y (sometimes another type of exposure) can only distort the association between the exposure of interest X and outcome Z, if it is associated with both X and Z. In the example, people who smoke tend to drink alcohol, and people who drink alcohol have a higher chance of developing cirrhosis.

Figure 1.1 The effect of an exposure on an outcome, with a third factor, the confounder.

Interest is only in the association between smoking (the exposure) and death from liver cirrhosis (the outcome); i.e. whether people who smoke have a higher chance of dying from cirrhosis than people who have never smoked.

In this hypothetical study, there are 1000 smokers and 1000 never-smokers.

(a)

	Current smokers	Never-smokers
Death rate from liver cirrhosis	15 per 1000	9 per 1000
% who drink alcohol	66	34

(b)

	Current smokers		Never-smokers	
	No. deaths/no. of men	Death rate per 1000 (A)	No. deaths/no. of men	Death rate per 1000 (B)
All	15/1000	15	9/1000	9
Non-drinkers	1/340	3	2/660	3
Drinkers	14/660	21	7/340	21

Figure 1.2 Hypothetical example of how a confounder can distort the results when examining the effect of an exposure on an outcome and how it can be allowed for.

This is shown in Figure 1.2b. By comparing the death rates between smokers and never-smokers <u>only</u> among non-drinkers, alcohol cannot have any confounding effect, because the two exposure groups have been 'made the same' in terms of alcohol consumption. The death rates are found to be identical, and the conclusion is reached that smoking is not associated with cirrhosis in this group. A similar finding is made among drinkers only, where, although the death rates are higher than those in non-drinkers (as expected), they are identical between smokers and never-smokers. The effect of confounding has been to create an association when really there was none. Analysing the data in this way (called a **stratified analysis**) is the simplest way to **allow** or **adjust for** a confounding factor. In practice, there are more efficient and sophisticated statistical methods to adjust for confounders (**regression analyses**; Chapter 4). If there is uncertainty over the relationship between the confounder and either the exposure or the outcome, it is worth taking it into account as a **potential confounding factor**.

A factor should not be considered a confounder if it lies on the same biological (causal) pathway between the exposure and an outcome [2]. For example, if looking at the effect of a high-fat diet on the risk of heart disease, high cholesterol is a consequence of the diet, and it can also lead to heart disease. Therefore, cholesterol would not be a confounder because it must, by definition, be causally associated with both exposure and outcome, and its effect should not (or cannot) be removed.

Bias
A **bias** occurs where the actions of participants or researchers produce a value of the study outcome measure that is *systematically* under- or over-reported in one group compared with another (i.e. it works in one direction). Figure 1.3 is a simple illustration. In the middle figure, only people who smoke lie about (misreport) their smoking status, and the effect of this is to **bias** the study result (in this case the prevalence of smoking). If, however, the number of non-smokers who lie about their smoking status is similar to that in smokers, even though there are lots of people who misreport their habits, the study result itself is not biased. But non-smokers rarely report themselves as smokers. It is important to focus on the bias in the *result* rather than the factor creating the bias.

Unlike confounding (where in the example above it was simple to obtain the alcohol status of the study subjects and, therefore, allow for it when examining the effect of smoking on liver cirrhosis), it is difficult to measure bias, because it would require the participants to admit whether or not they are lying, which, of course, would not happen. Researchers attempt to minimise bias at the design stage. In the example in Figure 1.3, estimating smoking prevalence could be assessed using biochemical confirmation of smoking status using nicotine or cotinine in the saliva of the participants, where high levels are indicative of being a smoker. However, even this is not perfect, because a light smoker could have low concentrations that overlap with non-smokers, and non-smokers heavily exposed to environmental tobacco smoke could have levels that overlap with some smokers. Many other biases are similarly difficult or impossible to measure.

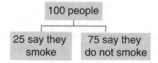

If no one has lied, then the true (and observed) prevalence of smoking is 25%. (25/100)

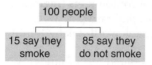

But if 10 of the 25 smokers lie <u>and</u> none of the non-smokers have lied, these 10 would be counted in the non-smoking group. The observed smoking prevalence would then be 15% (compared with the true value of 25%).

The study <u>result</u> would be **biased,** and **under-estimated.**

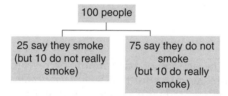

But if 10 of the smokers lie <u>and</u> 10 of the non-smokers have also lied, then although there are those who misreport their smoking status in both groups, the observed smoking prevalence would be 25% (the same as the true value).

The study <u>result</u> is not biased.

Figure 1.3 Illustration of bias, using an example in which the aim is to estimate the proportion of people who smoke, based on self-reported measures.

There are several types of biases (Box 1.6), and they can arise from something either the researcher or study participant has done [4]. To determine whether bias exists, the following questions should be considered:

• Was there anything unusual in how the participants were selected for the study?

• Were some participants managed, assessed, or examined differently from others?

• Is it plausible that certain participants could misreport, or under- or over-report, their responses to a questionnaire and hence distort the results?

1.3 Types of observational studies

Studies are conducted among two different types of participants:

1. **Population**: Participants are approached from the general population. They may or may not have the disorder of interest. Researchers sometimes

---

Box 1.6 Common types of potential biases

• **Selection bias**: The participants chosen for the study are not representative of the population of interest. An example is the healthy worker effect, where disease rates are lower in the study group than in the general population.
• **Response/responder (or non-response) bias**: People who agree to take part in a study have different characteristics from those who do not, and this distorts the results when making conclusions about the whole population.
• **Recall bias**: People with disease are often better at remembering past details (including past exposures) about their life than people without disease.
• **Withdrawal bias**: Participants who decide to discontinue with a study have different characteristics from those who continue, and this can distort the results because follow-up data (e.g. outcome measures) will be missing for some participants.
• **Assessment bias**: Different groups of participants are managed using different assessments or at different times according to their characteristics, exposure status, or health outcome.
• **Measurement bias**: Measuring exposures is performed differently for people with different health outcomes.
• **Observer or interviewer bias**: If an interviewer is aware of the participant's health (or other) status, this may influence the questions asked, or how they are asked, which consequently affects the response.

---

use the word **healthy** individual or **control** when describing some study participants, but this usually only means that the participants do not have the disorder of interest. They may have other disorders. Better terms could be **affected** and **unaffected**.
2. **Patients**: Only people who have already been diagnosed with a specific disorder are recruited to a study.

The study objectives are usually quite different for each of these two types. For studies of the **population**, interest is often in risk factors that lead to the occurrence of a disorder, but for **patient** studies interest could be in how an existing disorder develops including the management of it. Both can be used when describing characteristics of a group(s).

A variety of study designs can be used to examine associations, risk factors, and interventions.

• A **cross-sectional survey**: face-to-face interviews with participants or collecting self-completed participant surveys.
• A **(retrospective) case–control study**: people with and without a disorder of interest are identified and asked about their past habits, possibly also obtaining data from their medical records.
• A **prospective cohort study**: people without the disorder of interest are identified, baseline characteristics are measured, and participants are followed up for a period of time (several months or years) during which specific data is collected regularly.

- A **retrospective cohort study** is essentially a prospective cohort study that has already been conducted.
- **Longitudinal study**: a prospective cohort study in which exposures and often outcomes are measured repeatedly during follow-up.
- Studies based on routinely collected data: these could come from **regional or national registries or databases** (e.g. cancer or death notification systems) and contain a few key factors on each individual (e.g. age, sex, city of residence), as well as the disease status. Many such databases have adequate or good data quality processes in place, but a common limitation is that potential confounding factors are unavailable.

These terms for types of study designs should not be regarded as fixed. There may be occasions when one type could be used synonymously with another, a design is nested within another, or there are variations on a specific design. For example:

- There are nested case–control studies, which involve selecting and only analysing cases and controls (individuals with and without a disorder of interest) from a cohort study.
- Cases and controls could provide information about their current or past characteristics, but they might also be followed up for a certain length of time for other outcome measures, so these data are collected prospectively (similar to a prospective study).

Researchers simply need to be clear where the participants for a particular study have come from and how data are collected from or about them.

Large-scale studies could be preceded by a **pilot study** to examine the likely recruitment rate and how data are to be collected. Problems that arise can be dealt with before launching the full study. Pilot studies should have few participants and have a short duration.

An **ecological study** is one in which the unit of interest is a group of people, not an individual. For example, the relationship between income and risk of heart disease could be examined by using the average income from 20 countries and the corresponding rates of heart disease in each country, and then examine the correlation. However, such studies can often only provide a crude measure of association because potential unmeasured confounding factors could explain the effect (ecological fallacy); confounding is best dealt with at an individual level. The findings in ecological studies can therefore be inconsistent with those based on individuals.

A common but special type of observational study is a **qualitative research study**. This is usually based on relatively few participants (often < 50). Although a structured questionnaire could be used to ascertain some information about the participants, the main source of data is by face-to-face or telephone interviews, with largely open-ended questions to find out about their characteristics, lifestyle habits, opinions, or experiences (other study types almost always use structured questions). The interviews are usually recorded, allowing researchers to play back the recording later and code the responses in a way that can be interpreted and summarised. The findings are often descriptive, and the data produced cannot be readily quantified, and therefore not analysed using statistical methods covered in Chapter 4. For these reasons, they are not discussed in detail in this book, but they are well described elsewhere [5, 6]. A qualitative study can be used:

- As a precursor to the study designs mentioned previously in order to better design the questionnaires for a larger and more structured study (i.e. how to measure factors, exposures and outcomes), or to obtain an initial understanding of the research question
- To attempt clarification of some of the findings of studies, or a deeper understanding of them, especially if they are unexpected

Other types of observational studies include **case or case series reports**, which are based on unusual or sporadic occurrences found by a health professional, often during clinical practice [7]. They may provide interesting findings, but no firm conclusions should be made from these. They usually lead to better designed studies.

1.4 Strengths and limitations of the different types of study designs

There are ways of assessing the reliability of evidence from a particular study, such as the Grading of Recommendations Assessment, Development and Evaluation (GRADE) [8]. The most reliable type of study is, in order (generally, but there are exceptions):

- Systematic review of randomised clinical trials
- Individual randomised clinical trial
- Systematic review of observational studies
- Individual prospective cohort study
- Individual case–control study
- Individual cross-sectional study
- Hospital audits
- Case reviews

When examining risk factors and causality, there are many situations where a randomised trial cannot be conducted. For example, the best way to determine that smoking is a cause of cancer is to randomly allocate never-smokers to either take up smoking regularly for several years or remain non-smokers, then follow them up and compare the proportions that develop cancer between the two groups. This would clearly be unethical, so the only way to examine this risk factor is by using a cohort or case-control. Also, studies of aspects such as patient satisfaction and quality of care are generally descriptive, in which case a cross-sectional survey is the preferred method, because the primary purpose is not to look at the effect of an exposure on an outcome.

There can be some overlap between the different designs and more than one may be appropriate for a particular research question. A key distinction between them is **time**. Data can be collected retrospectively, from past participants/patients (hospital audits and case–control studies) or at one point in time, usually the present (cross-sectional studies). Alternatively, it can be collected prospectively, <u>after</u> entry to the study over a few months or several years, from newly identified participants/patients (cohort studies). It is also possible to conduct a retrospective cohort study, where data on exposures and outcomes have already been obtained, but there has still been a sufficient length of time between them. Such a study can be considered as a prospective study that has already been conducted.

Box 1.7 shows several strengths and limitations of different study designs, for consideration when choosing one over another. A cohort study is generally more reliable than a case–control study, but for uncommon disorder a cohort study conducted for several years that can only ascertain 50 cases is much less preferred than a case–control study in which 500 cases can be found quicker.

There is no such thing as the perfect study, regardless of how well it is designed. With hindsight, all investigators can identify ways in which their study could have been improved, having encountered problems and issue not expected at the start of the study that are associated with the design itself, data collection, and statistical analyses.

Observational studies for examining interventions
Observational studies have often been used to examine the efficacy or safety of an intervention [9], and they are a major feature of **comparative effectiveness research** [10–12]. However, there are design limitations that can produce a spurious or overestimated treatment effect (due to bias or confounding), and a randomised clinical trial is almost always preferred in this situation. Findings from observational studies can be consistent with those from randomised clinical trials (the gold standard for evaluating interventions). For example, a systematic review of 20 observational studies indicated that giving the influenza vaccine to the elderly could halve the risk of developing respiratory and flu-like symptoms [13], and the same effect was found in a large double-blind clinical trial [14].

A potential strength of observational studies, compared to randomised trials, is that they can provide supporting evidence for an intervention because the participants might be more representative of the target population (people who participate in clinical trials can sometimes be a self-selected group with different characteristics from those who decline to take part). Also, the study size is often larger than a clinical trial, making it easier to examine side effects, particularly those that are relatively uncommon.

However, there are situations where a treatment benefit has been found in observational studies, but not in a randomised clinical trial, or over-estimated or the opposite conclusion made. An example of the latter is where observational studies indicated that people with a high β-carotene intake (lots of fruit and vegetables) had a lower risk of cardiovascular death than those with a low intake (31% reduction in risk) [15], but randomised trials showed that a high intake might increase the risk by 12% [15].

1.5 Key design features

When conducting an observational study, there are several important design features to consider (covered in more detail in Chapters 5–8)
- Which study participants should be included (eligibility criteria)?
- Where will they come from (sampling frame)?

Box 1.7 Some strengths and limitations of the main observational study designs

Study design	Strengths	Limitations
Cross-sectional survey (retrospective).	• Can be inexpensive and quick to conduct • Can estimate prevalence of a disorder or event. • Usually no concept of loss to follow-up (i.e. participants who drop out of the study). • Can examine several exposures and several outcomes.	• Response rates may be low, leading to problems selection or responder bias. • Recall bias can be a problem if participants are asked about past information. • If examining an intervention, it may not be possible to ascertain from records why some patients received the intervention and others did not. • Can only examine association between an exposure and outcome (not causality).
Case–control study (retrospective).	• Can be relatively inexpensive and quick to conduct. • Suitable for studying rare disorders or events. • Usually no concept of loss to follow-up. • Can examine several exposures in relation to a single disorder.	• Not suitable for studying uncommon exposures. • Could be affected by recall and selection biases. • Not possible to determine prevalence or incidence of disease. • It can sometimes be difficult to establish whether the exposure came before the outcome (required for causality). • Care is required when selecting cases and controls (i.e. that they both come from the target population of interest).
Prospective cohort study.	• Prospective follow-up means that exposures and outcome measures should be easier to record. • Can estimate the incidence of a disease. • Possible to look at how exposure changes over time. • Less chance of selection or recall bias. • It is known that the exposure came before the outcome (required for causality). • Can examine the natural history of a disorder. • Can examine several disorders in relation to a single exposure. • Can examine several exposures in relation to a single outcome.	• Can be expensive, both in terms of money and staff resources. • Can take a long time before final results are available. • Not suitable for investigating rare disorders or events. • If the exposure status changes over time, this needs to be ascertained, and the statistical analyses are more complex. • Potentially many participants could drop out (especially with long follow-up), so there would be no measure of the study endpoints on these. • If the characteristics of those who drop out are very different between the exposed and unexposed groups, this could create bias. • Could be affected by non-response and time-related biases.

Retrospective cohorts have similar features to prospective ones, except they are relatively inexpensive but can be affected by missing data.

- What will be done to them, and how often (collecting data)?
- How will the exposures, confounding factors, and outcome measures be measured?
- How will potential confounding and bias be minimised or addressed?

Eligibility criteria and recruitment

In many observational studies, the study population should be defined by a set of **inclusion and exclusion criteria**. They specify which participants are recruited or whose data to include (if the study is based on patient medical records or established databases). Each subject has to meet the criteria before being included in the study, though there may be acceptable small deviations. The criteria depend on the research objectives, and may include an age range and the ability to provide informed consent. Eligibility criteria should have unambiguous definitions to make recruiting participants easier. Some studies, such as those based only on patient records, might have few or no criteria, because they are based on every patient with a certain disorder.

Determining the eligibility criteria necessitates balancing the advantages and disadvantages of having a highly selected group against those associated with including a wide variety of participants. Having many narrow criteria (e.g. age range of 30–35) produces a group in which there should be relatively little variability ('make everything the same'), and it is easier to find associations especially if the effect is small or moderate. However, the study results may not be easily generalisable. A study with few criteria that are wide (e.g. age ≥18) will have a more general application, but the amount of variability could make it more difficult to detect an association, and sometimes only large effects can be found easily.

Not everyone who is eligible for a particular study will agree to participate, and the higher the acceptance rate, the better. However, if, for example, more than 40% decline to take part, it can be useful to attempt to obtain some information from these participants (e.g. characteristics such as age, gender, and some measure of the exposure factor), which can be used to compare with those who agreed to participate. The study results could be biased if those who refused and those who participated are very different. Reasons for non-participation could also be used to redesign parts of the study while it is being conducted to improve uptake.

Encouraging patients to take part in a clinical trial of a treatment may be easier than an observational study, because they see a potential personal benefit, assuming the treatment is effective. However, this is not the case for observational studies, so maximising uptake is worthwhile (Box 1.8).

Sampling frame

A key design feature of all observational studies is the **sampling frame**. This is a list of people from which the target group of interest will be identified. It is essentially the starting point of a study. There are many examples of sampling frames; they can be local to the researchers, where access is easy (e.g.

Box 1.8 Possible ways of encouraging people to take part in an observational study (if it involves recruiting people)

• Make clear what the potential benefits are to society and possibly themselves (e.g. identifying new lifestyle risk factors that individuals can modify after the study results are available)
• Minimise inconvenience associated with collecting data and measuring exposures and outcomes
• Provide costs to cover travel and subsistence if the study involves attending clinics for assessments
• Provide information about or discuss possible anxieties people may have about health issues to be raised by the study

---

people registered at a single physician's practice or listed outpatients in a single hospital respiratory clinic); **regional** (e.g. all adults listed on the census or registry in a town or geographical region or found using telephone directories); or **national** (e.g. all registered general practitioners in England, access to adults listed on all censuses or registries in a country, or a register for a specific disorder).

The choice of sampling frame (local, regional, or national) will depend on the research question and how representative the research results need to be. Examples of sampling frames and research objectives are given in chapters 5–8, and they should allow the conclusions of the study to be generalisable to the wider population of interest. For example, a study of factors that influence the severity of chronic obstructive lung disease (COPD) could be conducted in a respiratory clinic at a hospital, but this would exclude COPD cases who only see their family physician and may therefore have milder disease. Also, researchers use local sampling frames because they have limited staff or funds.

Once the sampling frame has been determined, the next question is whether to include everyone within it or a **random sample**. This choice, again, is influenced by costs and feasibility. If a random sample is used, the process should be explicitly described, and there are various methods for appropriately selecting participants at random, to help to ensure that some participants are not chosen in a way that could produce a bias [16].

Collecting data

All observational studies involve collecting data, which may or may not require direct input from the study participants. There are several ways in which this could be done (Box 1.9). Different sources of data have different attributes, such as quality, validity, reliability, and measurement error [17]. Obtaining information directly from participants will be a choice between interviews or self-completed questionnaires, and each has strengths and limitations (Box 1.10). Missing data is a major problem that usually cannot be

---

Box 1.9 Sources of data within observational studies

• Face-to-face or telephone interviews directly with study participants.
• Self-completed questionnaires (handed or posted back to the researchers), including self-completed diaries.
• Face-to-face interviews or questionnaires completed by a proxy for the study participant (e.g. close relative or friend).
• Biological samples (e.g. blood, urine, saliva, or tissue).
• Imaging tests (e.g. X-ray, CT, or MRI scan) or clinical examinations.
• Environmental measures (e.g. air pollution, quality of drinking water).
• Health records from family or primary care clinics or hospitals.
• Local, regional, or national registries/database that routinely record population data on, for example, deaths and cause of death, occurrence of cancer, occurrence of specific disorders, or hospital admissions. Study participants would need to be **linked** to these databases using personal identifiers.

These methods could be used on their own or in combination for a particular study.

Box 1.10 Strengths and limitations of obtaining information from study participants using either interview or self-completed questionnaires

Interview	Self-completed questionnaire
Requires dedicated staff to meet with each participant at their home or a research site, or to interview by telephone (can therefore be expensive)	Can be sent out and received by post, allowing a wider coverage of the sampling frame (can therefore be relatively inexpensive)
Direct contact encourages participants to respond and to complete most/all questions	Can be affected by moderate to high non-response rates and missing data for several questions
Complex questions misunderstood by the participant could be clarified by the interviewer	Complex questions can be difficult to interpret. This can be helped using clear instructions on how to complete these questionnaire fields
Interviewer may have limited time to spend with each participant, so the questionnaire should be relatively short	Participant can complete the questionnaire in their own time and therefore more questions could be included
Useful when responses to some questions need probing or further clarification	Useful for questionnaires containing sensitive questions, including those that require anonymity
Interviewers could influence (bias) the responses, particularly if they are aware of the participant's exposure or disease status and are aware of the study objectives	The researchers cannot directly influence the responses

overcome with most retrospective studies, but attempts could be made to minimise this in prospective studies by using good data collection systems (e.g. simple/short questionnaires; see Box 5.6). Also, regular (e.g. yearly) general updates of the study to all participants could keep them interested, minimising dropouts (and therefore withdrawal bias).

A prospective cohort study is generally the only type of observational study that usually involves collecting data directly from participants over time. This is often done using questionnaires, but some studies might involve physical and clinical examinations, and collection of biological samples or imaging tests. A **schedule of assessments** must be drawn up, stating explicitly when contact is to be made with the participants and how data are to be collected at each time point. A vital part of follow-up is the evaluation of the outcome measure, which may be done through regular reviews of clinic records or by linking the study participants to regional or national registries that routinely collect information on disease occurrence or deaths.

With advances in information technology, more people now have personal computers, mobile telephones, or smartphones, and observational studies will probably make use of these. Study participants could complete question-naires online (rather than face-to-face with a researcher) or by using a Personal Digital Assistant provided by the researchers specifically for the study. These approaches have the potential advantages of targeting a wider and more gen-eralisable population (larger sampling frame), increasing response rates, and decreasing study costs (reduced central data management because there will be much less data to be entered manually). Key considerations in dealing with these advances will be that such studies may only be tenable in countries where many/most people have access to personal computers, and there may be issues over representativeness (whether characteristics differ significantly between people who do and do not have a computer) and security (accessing a central research database and exchanging sensitive patient confidential data that require the anonymity of the participant.)

Studies using only patient medical records

Patient medical records (from hospitals, family physicians or registries) are sometimes used as the only source of data for observational studies. This is particularly useful when there is limited time, because the data already exist and nothing is required from patients directly. However, such studies are almost always based on patients seen in routine practice, so researchers can only use data that have already been collected. Data can be clinical, blood or imaging measurements, pathology results, or standard characteristics such as sex, age, ethnic origin, and disease status.

Observational studies that use stored records usually consist of people who already have a disorder or are seeking professional health care, instead of individuals from a general 'healthy' population. Therefore, a common objec-tive is to provide simple descriptive statistics on a defined group of patients, or to examine an intervention or a care pathway. They can also be used to investigate associations or prognostic markers.

Box 1.11 Key characteristics of studies according to method of data collection

Manual extraction	Electronic data systems
The person extracting the data may form a reasonable view of general aspects of the data such as quality	Can provide a large number of patients
Potentially important factors/measurements that had not been originally planned could be identified and collected during data extraction	Selecting patients, using the predefined eligibility criteria, could be more accurate
Given limited resources, only one or few searches of the records could be made	Multiple searches of the database can be made easily

---

Choosing which patients to include involves specifying clear and simple selection criteria, and a time frame (e.g. all newly diagnosed cases of thyroid cancer between 1995 and 2012). Too many selection criteria could limit the number of patient records for the study. However, the main problems are missing data and data quality (inconsistencies cannot usually be clarified nor errors corrected).

Older data, from patients seen many years ago, are more likely to be stored on paper (in the clinic, or may have to be retrieved from an off-site archive). Extracting such data can be laborious, requiring staff to examine each patient record and manually transfer the factors (variables) of interest onto a study data sheet. All of the factors should be pre-specified, to avoid staff having to conduct repeated searches and extractions of the same patient records. Many health service providers now use electronic patient data systems, and it may appear relatively simple to download a set of specific variables for a defined group of patients. However, many clinical IT systems were not set up for research purposes, so downloading data may require a dedicated programmer. IT support may also be required to collect and merge data from several clinics, especially if they use different software systems. Some key characteristics of manually extracting data or obtaining it from electronic databases are shown in Box 1.11.

Clear definition of the exposures and outcome measures

The key factors (variables) of interest in a study, especially those that involve examining the effects of exposures on outcome measures, require clear definitions as do all potential confounding factors. Having well-defined endpoints and objectives will facilitate:
- Conduct of the study (e.g. the researchers are focussed)
- Decisions on what data (information) to collect and how to do this

- Analysis of the data
- Interpretation of the results
- Writing of the final report for publication

It will also help to reduce significant criticism of the paper when submitted for publication in a peer-reviewed journal, acknowledging that there may not be perfect (standard) definitions of either the exposures or the outcomes, and some may disagree with a chosen definition. The key factors should be measured objectively, rather than subjectively, where possible (e.g. measuring carbon monoxide in exhaled breath versus self-report in a study of smokers who quit).

Many exposures may initially appear easy to define, but on closer inspection they often have several descriptions. For example, if examining the effect of alcohol consumption habits on emergency hospital admissions for physical injuries, 'alcohol drinking' could be measured as any of the following:

- Someone who regularly drinks alcohol (i.e. at least once per week)
- Number of units drunk in previous week
- Number of units drunk over a typical month

Ideally, outcomes (such as disorders) should be measured using standard and generally accepted methods, (e.g. histopathology for cancer) or established diagnostic tools (e.g. *Diagnostic and Statistical Manual of Mental Disorders* for psychological disorders).

In this book, a variety of exposures and outcomes are used as examples. It is useful to realise that they can be analysed and interpreted in a similar way:

- Clinical features or characteristics
- Environmental exposures
- Lifestyle habits or characteristics
- Imaging marker
- Biomarker
- Intervention
- Perceived experiences and measures of satisfaction

Consideration of confounding and bias

Information on known and potentially important confounding factors should be collected as part of the study. In a study of long duration, it might be possible to add 'new' confounding factors to the **case report forms** at a later date (see Chapter 11, page 226).

Taking account of the common types of bias (Box 1.6) can usually help to design the study to avoid or minimise the effects, though this is sometimes difficult:

- Careful selection of study participants, without choosing them on the basis of factors of interest, can minimise selection bias, for example, not trying to recruit heavier smokers for a study of the association between smoking and a disorder.
- Where possible, objective measures of exposures and outcomes should be used.
- Where possible, have an independent review of the outcome measures, ideally where the reviewer is blind to (i.e. unaware of) the exposure status of the participants.

1.6 Interpreting and reporting the results and implication for public health or clinical practice

A major task for the investigators is to analyse and interpret the findings, and communicate the results through conferences and journal articles. The following structure will be used in Chapters 5–7, in the sections entitled 'Analysing data and interpreting results'.

What are the main results?
It is important to focus on the main result(s) in the context of the study objectives. Researchers should examine this first and ensure they understand this (quantitatively), including clinical importance and any implications.

What could the true effect be, given that the study was conducted on a sample of people?
After the main result(s) have been interpreted, it is necessary to examine **95% confidence intervals** (90 or 99% are alternatives), because these will provide a likely range of the *true* effect (see Chapter 3).

Could the observed result be a chance finding in this particular study?
Statistical significance (p-values) is a useful part of the analyses, but it is important to understand them fully, including what influences the size of a p-value (see Chapter 3).

How good is the evidence?
Considering major strengths and limitations of a study and the study findings is essential, including whether the findings and conclusions are generalisable. Also, whether the interpretation of the findings is likely to have been influenced by bias or confounding. If there were significant confounding factors or bias, is the main result unreliable? No individual study should change practice. There should always be corroborating evidence from at least one other study, and this can include:
- Other similar studies (same exposure and similar population)
- Studies of the same exposure in different populations
- Studies investigating the biological plausibility, including laboratory evidence (i.e. whether the association makes sense)

Finally, researchers should always attempt to suggest what should happen next, and discuss how the main findings and conclusions of their study should be used, for example, to change clinical or public health practice or to make recommendations for further research.

1.7 Translational research

It is becoming increasingly common to collect biological specimens as part of the main study, to be stored centrally in a laboratory for either pre-specified analyses to be performed at the end of the study, or for future as yet unspecified

---

Box 1.12 Some key considerations for studies examining biomarkers

• A central laboratory should be used, unless the marker is well-established and commercial assays are available.
• Good systems must be in place for collecting, processing, and shipping biological samples, for all recruiting centres and the central laboratory.
• If the samples are obtained from many study participants, across many centres (including serial samples over time from the same participant), there should be (electronic) systems for tracking the samples from the centre to the central laboratory.
• Secure and well-maintained storage of samples should be set up, e.g. fridges or freezers, with proper labelling and coding of each sample allowing it to be retrieved easily, and matched (anonymously) to the correct study participant. Electronic barcode readers could be useful when there are many samples, because this reduces human coding errors. Also, the storage facilities (e.g. freezer/fridge temperature) should be monitored continuously.
• Quality control processes should be in place continuously (this might include repeated measurements of the same samples).
• The laboratory assay or technique to measure the marker should have been validated, and error/failure rates examined, including measurement error.
• Semi-automated or manual assessment (scoring) of samples needs clear specification, and ideally. each sample (or a random subset) needs to be assessed by two independent people.
• Should tissue be collected from people with or without a disorder of interest, or disease/damaged and healthy tissue from the same persons.

---

analyses. This will involve the creation and maintenance of a **biobank**. The samples are usually blood, saliva, or urine, but may also include tissue samples (e.g. cancerous tissue removed from affected patients). The analyses involve measuring biomarkers, which could be chemical or biological (e.g. genetic or protein markers), or imaging markers, and these are correlated with clinical outcomes from the main study, such as the risk of disease, disease severity, or mortality. Many biological or imaging factors can be analysed like traditional (external) exposures.

One of the main purposes of these analyses is to examine the prognostic value of a marker, that is, how well it **predicts** a clinical outcome (Chapter 8). A key issue is the reliability of a marker and that it has been properly validated (i.e. it measures what it is meant to measure). Box 1.12 shows important features of biomarker studies.

Not all studies will benefit from having a translational study component, and indeed the collection and storage of biological samples could sometimes be a hindrance to the main study, by adding significant extra financial costs and time to collect the samples. Researchers should decide whether translational research is essential for their study.

Biological samples could be used to examine:
- The relationship between the biomarker and an exposure (e.g. lifestyle, environmental, or clinical characteristics)
- The relationship between the biomarker and a disorder (or other event)
- Methods for detecting or diagnosing disease
- Methods for detecting infectious or microbial agents
- Biological mechanisms and processes
- Surveillance (or monitoring) within a population

This field of work can be called **molecular epidemiology** [18].

When using biological samples, it is important that enough material is collected for the study objectives, and this should be agreed with the laboratory staff (e.g. minimum amount of blood). Also, how the samples are to be handled, for example, stored at room temperature or in fridge or freezer, and whether samples need to be posted immediately by courier or in batches.

1.8 Key points

- Natural variability or variation underpins aspects of study design and analysis.
- Observational studies can be used to describe the characteristics of a single group of people.
- Another major purpose is to examine the effect of an exposure on an outcome.
- To do this reliably, we need to make the exposed group 'the same' as the unexposed group (except the exposure factor of interest).
- Confounding and bias are the most common reasons why the exposure groups are not 'the same'.
- There are several types of observational studies, each with strengths and limitations: cross-sectional, case–control, and retrospective or prospective cohort.
- All studies need clear definitions of factors, exposures, and outcomes.
- Reliable processes should be in place for dealing with biological specimens for translational research.

References

1. Silman AJ, Macfarlane GJ. *Epidemiological Studies: A Practical Guide*. Cambridge University Press. Second Edition (2002).
2. Rothman KJ. *Epidemiology: An Introduction*. Oxford University Press. First Edition (2002).
3. Barker DJP, Rose G. *Epidemiology in Medical Practice*. Churchill Livingstone. Fourth Edition 1990.
4. Grimes DA, Schulz KF. Bias and causal associations in observational studies. *Lancet* 2002;359:248–52.
5. Pope C, Mays N. *Qualitative Research in Health Care*. Wiley-Blackwell. Third Edition. (2006).
6. Silverman D. *Doing Qualitative Research: A Practical Handbook*. SAGE Publications. Fourth Edition (2013).

7. Grimes DA, Schulz KF. Descriptive studies: what they can and cannot do. *Lancet* 2002;359: 145–9

8. http://www.gradeworkinggroup.org/index.htm. Accessed 14 May 2014.

9. MacMahon S, Collins R. Reliable assessment of the effects of treatment on mortality and major morbidity, II: observational studies. *Lancet* 2001;357:455–62

10. Sox HC, Goodman SN. The methods of comparative effectiveness research. *Annu Rev Public Health* 2012;33:425–45.

11. Armstrong K. Methods in comparative effectiveness research. *J Clin Oncol* 2012;30:4208–14

12. Korn EL, Freidlin B. Methodology for comparative effectiveness research: potential and limitations. *J Clin Oncol* 2012;30:4185–7.

13. Gross PA, Hermogenes H, Sacks HS, Lau J, Levandowski RA. The efficacy of influenza vaccine in elderly persons. *Ann Intern Med* 1995;123:518–27.

14. Govaert TME, Thijs MCN, Masurel N, Sprenger MJW, Dinant GJ, Knottnerus JA. The efficacy of influenza vaccination in elderly individuals. *JAMA* 1994;272(21):1661–5

15. Egger M, Schneider M, Davey SG. Spurious precision? Meta-analysis of observational studies. *BMJ*. 1998;316(7125):140–4

16. Moser C, Kalton G. *Survey Methods in Social Investigation*. Dartmouth Publishing Co. Second Edition (1985)

17. dos Santos Silva I. Measurement of exposures and outcomes. In: *Cancer Epidemiology: Principles and Methods*. IARC Press (1999). http://www.iarc.fr/en/publications/pdfs-online/epi/cancerepi/. Accessed 14 May 2014.

18. Rothman N, Hainaut P, Schulte P, Smith M, Boffetta P, Perera F, eds. *Molecular Epidemiology: Principles and Practices*. International Agency for Research on Cancer (IARC) (2011).

CHAPTER 2

Outcome measures, risk factors, and causality

This chapter describes the three fundamental types of measurements used in observational studies and how data based on each type are summarised and introduces the concepts of risk and risk factors and how evidence for a causal link between an exposure and outcome measure could be determined.

2.1 Types of measurements (endpoints)

All observational studies involve collecting data from or about participants. The data may include many factors (or variables), such as demographic information, data about current or past lifestyle and habits, physical or psychological symptoms, or biochemical or imaging markers. To make sense of a dataset and to communicate the findings, it is essential to summarise the data in a quantitative and objective way [1–3]. For example, a study conclusion that 'smoking is very bad for you' is easy to read, but provides no useful information. The word 'very' is highly subjective. What does 'bad for you' mean? Is it an increased risk of the following:

- Developing cancer
- Dying from lung cancer
- Developing cardiovascular disease
- Dying from any cause

To describe a set of characteristics among a group of people, or examine relationships between exposures and outcomes, requires four key stages:

1. Identifying an appropriate endpoint (that can be measured and quantified), as well as other factors of interest (that can also be quantified)
2. Obtaining data from every participant in the study, who will have at least one measure of the outcome(s), as well as values for all the other factors
3. Summarising these data (i.e. turning many data values into one or a few)
4. Interpreting the summary results

A Concise Guide to Observational Studies in Healthcare, First Edition. Allan Hackshaw.
© 2015 John Wiley & Sons, Ltd. Published 2015 by John Wiley & Sons, Ltd.

Box 2.1   Types and examples of outcome measures

After defining a health outcome, in what way is the unit of interest (person) evaluated in order to measure the outcome?

Counting people: individuals are put into mutually exclusive groups, based on a specified characteristic, and we count how many have a specified event (binary/ categorical data)

Dead or alive
Suffered a first heart attack (yes or no)
Recovered from disease (yes or no)
Severity of disease (mild, moderate, severe)
Ability to perform household duties (none, a little, some, moderate, high)
Has specific genetic mutation or not

Taking measurements on people (continuous data), measuring a characteristic or biological endpoint (individuals are not divided into mutually exclusive groups)

Age at diagnosis of a disorder
Body weight
Cholesterol level
Number of days in hospital
Number of units of alcohol intake per week
Quality of life score

Time-to-event: measuring the time taken until a specified event occurs*. This category is essentially a combination of the previous two categories - there is a defined event (counting people) and a length of time (taking measurements on people).

Time until death
Time until the occurrence of a heart attack or stroke
Time until discharged from hospital

*all study participants without the event are 'censored', see page 31

Summarising data is achieved by classifying the type of measurement into one of three possible categories, after first determining the **unit of interest**. In observational studies this is almost always a single individual (person).[#] Consideration is then given to the way in which the unit of interest (i.e. person) will be evaluated when measuring the endpoint or factor. The three categories are:
- counting people
- taking measurements on people
- measuring the time until an event occurs (time-to-event)
Box 2.1 defines these groups, and shows examples.

[#] In ecological studies, the unit of interest is a group of individuals from a single geographical location (e.g. town, region, or country), but only summary data from the group is available, often from national or international statistics.

Knowing into which of the three categories the outcome measure of interest falls is essential for:
- Helping define the study objectives
- Designing the study (e.g. the method of sample size estimation)
- Analysing the data (choosing an appropriate statistical method)
- Interpreting the results

In a study of the effect of an exposure on an outcome, the *exposure* is usually categorised as 'counting people' or 'taking measurements on people'; it is unusual (statistically difficult) to have an exposure that involves time-to-event data, unless they have all had the event, in which case the measure can be treated as a continuous factor.

There are established statistical methods for analysing each type of outcome measure. The more simple methods can examine the effect of only one exposure on one outcome measure, each measured only once, but more powerful methods (regression analyses) can allow examination of several exposures, or one exposure and several confounding factors (see Chapter 4).

Sections 2.2 to 2.4 introduce the three categories of outcome measures when considering a single group of people, and researchers should always consider how to display data in a diagram. Further details of how some of the statistics are calculated are found elsewhere [1-3]; the focus here is on interpretation. To investigate associations, comparisons are made between *two or more groups*, covered in Chapter 3.

2.2 'Counting people' (risk)

This type of outcome measure is easily summarised by calculating the **percentage** or **proportion**. For example, the prevalence of smokers among a group of individuals is found by counting how many people smoke, and dividing this number by the total number of individuals. When examining disorders, the proportion can be called **risk**, and the simplest calculation is the number of individuals with the disorder divided by the total number in the group. Risk and risk factors are described in more detail in Section 2.6. 'Counting people' endpoints can be shown diagrammatically using a **bar chart** (e.g. Figures 5.1 and 5.2).

2.3 'Taking measurements on people'

Whereas data based on 'counting people' endpoints can be summarised by a single parameter (proportion), taking measurements on people requires two parameters: **typical value** and **spread** (some measure of how much the outcome varies between people). The following cholesterol levels (mmol/L) for 40 healthy men are ranked in order of size:

3.6	3.8	3.9	4.1	4.2	4.5	4.5	4.8	5.1	5.3
5.4	5.4	5.6	5.8	5.9	6.0	6.1	6.1	6.2	6.3
6.4	6.5	6.6	6.8	6.9	7.1	7.2	7.2	7.3	7.4
7.5	7.7	8.0	8.1	8.1	8.2	8.3	9.0	9.1	10.0

A typical value, the 'average' or measure of central tendency, is where the middle of the distribution lies. Two measures are:
- **Mean**: sum of all the values, divided by the number of observations (in the example, $256/40 = 6.4$ mmol/L)
- **Median**: the value that has half the observations above it and half below, when ranked in order of size (in the example, it is halfway between the 20th and 21st, $(6.3 + 6.4)/2 = 6.35$ mmol/L)

Some men will have a cholesterol value below 6.4, some above, and some exactly 6.4, but the *average* is 6.4 mmol/L. The mean or median cannot describe the whole range of values. Therefore using a single summary number to help interpret the data will be imperfect, but makes it easier to interpret the data.

Two measures of spread are:
- **Standard deviation**: the amount of variability, i.e. how much the data spreads from the mean. In the example, it is 1.57 mmol/L: the cholesterol levels differ from the mean value of 6.4 by, *on average*, 1.57 mmol/L.
- **Interquartile range**: the difference between the 25th centile (the value that has a quarter of the data below it and three-quarters above it) and the 75th centile (the value that has three-quarters of the data below it and a quarter above it). In the example, it is $7.47 - 5.32 = 2.15$ mmol/L. Sometimes, it is more useful just to present the actual 25th and 75th centiles.

'Taking measurements on people' endpoints can be shown diagrammatically using **scatter plots** (see Figure 4.1, and also Figure 5.3).

Deciding which measures of average and spread to use depends on whether or not the distribution is symmetric. To determine this, the data can be grouped into categories of cholesterol levels, to produce a **frequency distribution**, and the percentage (proportion) in each group are used to create a **histogram** (the shaded boxes in Figure 2.1). The shape is reasonably symmetric, indicating that the distribution is **Gaussian** or **Normal**[#], which is more easily visualised by drawing a bell-shaped curve (Figure 2.1).

When data are Normally distributed, the mean and median are similar, and the preferred measures of average and spread are the mean and standard deviation, because they have useful mathematical properties which underlie many statistical methods used to analyse this type of data. When the data are not Normally distributed, the median and interquartile range are better measures.

Distributions can be **positively skewed** or skewed to the right, where the tail of the data is (i.e. the values are 'bunched' up towards the lower end of the range); or **negatively skewed**, when the tail of the data is towards the left. The mean and median will be very different, but the median is usually a better measure of a typical value. When data are skewed, transformations may make the distribution approximately Normal (symmetric): logarithms, square root or reciprocal (positive skew), or square or cubic (negatively skew). Many biological measurements only have a Normal distribution after the

---

[#] 'N' is in capital letters to avoid confusion with the usual definition of the word normal, which can indicate people without disease

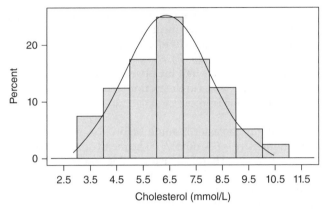

Figure 2.1 Histogram of the cholesterol values in 40 men, with a superimposed Normal (Gaussian) distribution curve.

logarithm is taken. The mean is calculated on the log of the values, and the result is back-transformed to the original scale, though this cannot be done with standard deviation. Negative skewed data could also be 'reflected': subtract them all from the largest value then add one (making the distribution positively skewed), and then apply logarithms. Sometimes there is no transformation that will turn a skewed distribution into a reasonably Normal one.

A reliable approach for assessing Normality is examining a **probability** (or **centile**) **plot**[#], which statistical software packages can easily provide. There are various versions, but the only aspect that matters is that the observations lie *reasonably* along a straight line, if the data are approximately Normally distributed (some curvature, or a few outliers at either end are often acceptable).

2.4 Time-to-event data

As with 'counting people' endpoints, an 'event' needs to be defined for time-to-event data. The simplest and most commonly used is 'death', hence the term **survival analysis**. In the following seven participants, the endpoint is "time from baseline until death, in years", and all seven participants have died:

4.5   6.1   6.7   8.3   9.1   9.4   10.0

The mean (7.7 years) and median (8.3 years) are easily calculated (as with 'taking measurements on people'). However, in another group of nine participants, not all have died at the time of statistical analysis:

2.7   2.9   3.3   4.7   5.1   6.8   7.2   7.8   9.1
dead   dead   alive   dead   alive   alive   dead   dead   alive

---

[#] Medical statistics books can provide a technical description of how the plot is obtained, but here we cover how to interpret it

Here, the mean or median cannot be calculated in the usual way, until all the participants have died, which could take many years. Calculating the average time until death by ignoring those who are still alive is incorrect; the summary measure would be biased downwards because insufficient time has elapsed for the others to die, after which the average time to death would be longer. Alternatively, we could obtain the survival rate at a designated point. Among the 9 people, two died before 3 years and 7 lived beyond, so the 3-year survival rate is $7/9 = 78\%$. This is then simply an example of 'counting people'. Every participant would need to be followed up for at least 3 years, unless they died, and the outcome (dead or alive) must be known at that point for all participants. There are two main problems: (i) losing contact with some participants, particularly after long follow up, and (ii) this approach does not distinguish between someone who died at 2 months from another person who died at 2.5 years.

A better approach is to use a **life-table**, which produces a **Kaplan-Meier curve**. In the example above, the 'time from baseline until death or last known to be alive' is one variable, and another variable has values 0 or 1 to indicate 'still alive' or 'dead'. Someone who is still alive (i.e. not had the event of interest), or last known to be alive at a certain date, is said to be **censored**. This approach uses the last available information on every participant, and allows for how long he/she has lived, or has been in the study.

Table 2.1 is the life table for the group of nine participants above, and the first and last columns are plotted to produce the Kaplan-Meier curve in Figure 2.2. When each participant dies, the step drops down. The four censored participants contribute no further information to the analysis after the date when they were last known to be alive. It is possible to estimate two

Table 2.1 Life table for the survival data of nine participants on page 30.

Time since diagnosis (years)	Censored (0 = yes, 1 = dead)	Number of participants at risk	Percentage alive (survival rate %)*
0	—	9	100
2.7	1	9	89
2.9	1	8	78
3.3	0	7	78
4.7	1	6	65
5.1	0	5	65
6.8	0	4	65
7.2	1	3	43
7.8	1	2	22
9.1	1	1	22

*The chance of being alive at a certain time point, given that the person has survived up to that point; calculated using a formula [1].
• To obtain the 4-year survival rate from the table, it is necessary to ascertain whether there is a value at exactly 4 years. Because there is none, the closest value from below is taken, that is, at 3.3 years: 4-year survival rate is 78%.
   To obtain the median survival, the point at which 50% of study participants are alive is determined. The closest value from below is 43%, so the median is 7.2 years.

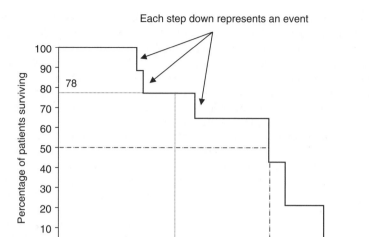

Figure 2.2 Kaplan–Meier plot of the survival data for the nine participants on page 30, which can also be used to estimate survival rates and median survival:
4-year survival rate: A vertical line is drawn on the x-axis at 4, and the rate is the corresponding y-axis value where the line hits the curve, that is, 78%.
Median survival: The time at which half the participants have died. A horizontal line is drawn on the y-axis at 50%, and the corresponding x-axis value (median) is where the line hits the curve, that is, 7.2 years.

summary measures from Figure 2.2 or Table 2.1: **median survival**, and a **survival rate at a specific time point**. Median survival is reliable when many events have occurred, fairly continuously, throughout the study; otherwise it can be skewed by only one or two events. Sometimes, an event (survival) rate at a specific time point is preferred.

When all participants have had the event of interest (such as death), the Kaplan-Meier median survival will be the same as the simple median from a ranked list of numbers. The two medians are only different when some participants are censored (i.e. not had the event). The median is used instead of the mean, because time-to-event data often has a skewed distribution.

The usual Kaplan-Meier plot has a vertical (y) axis which represents the *event-free rate* (e.g. survival), so the curve starts at 100% at time zero. This is useful when events (here deaths) tend to occur early in the study. However, the plot could instead have a vertical axis that represents the *event rate*, so the curve starts at 0% at time zero (i.e. it uses 100 minus the fourth column in Table 2.2). This type of plot may be more informative when events tend to occur later on. A curve based on the *event-free* rate must start at 100% at time zero, but because the y-axis for a plot showing the *event* rate starts at zero, the upper limit can be less than 100%.

Different types of time-to-event outcome measures

In the section above, the 'event' in the time-to-event endpoint is 'death', sometimes called **overall survival** (OS), because it relates to death from any cause. It is simple because it only requires the date of death. The methods can apply to any endpoint that involves measuring the time until a specified event has occurred, for example, time from entry to a study until the occurrence or recurrence of a disorder or any change in health status, such as time until hospital discharge. Two other common measures associated with the risk of a disorder are:

- **Cause-specific survival**: the event is death due to a specific disorder, and all other deaths and participants who are still alive are censored. This requires, in addition to date of death, accurate confirmation of cause of death (such as pathology records), which is not always reliably recorded.
- **Event-free survival** (EFS) or **disease-free survival** (DFS): the event can be one of several disorders, and only participants who have not had any of the events and not died are censored. For example, in studies of cardiovascular disease, an event could be one of four types: fatal or non-fatal coronary heart disease, or fatal or non-fatal stroke. Only the time until the first event has occurred is taken, because afterwards the person may be managed or treated differently, making it difficult to distinguish whether subsequent events are attributable to the exposures of interest or management/treatment.

When considering OS, DFS or EFS, the terminology implies that interest is in those who survive (i.e. do not have the event of interest). However, the analysis and interpretation focus on the event itself (mortality or the event/disorder).

2.5 What could the true effect be, given that the study was conducted on a sample of people?

The traditional approach in medical research studies is to consider the concept of a **true effect**. For a single group of individuals, this could be a true proportion, mean value, median survival time, or event rate at a specific time point. As an example, in a cross-sectional study of UK vocational dental practitioners (VDP) (see Box 5.2 and Table 5.1), there was a finite number (n = 767) of individuals in the population in 2005, and one aim was to examine their alcohol habits. If every single VDP responded to the survey, and did so truthfully, this would give the true prevalence of alcohol use without uncertainty. However, of the 767 registered VDPs, 502 responded, so there will be uncertainty over the habits among the 265 who did not.

The original study research question is fundamental. In the VDP study, this was 'What is the prevalence of smoking, alcohol, and recreational drug use among all UK VDPs in 2005?'. The word all is key. Because the study aimed to observe all UK VDPs, inferences about the 767 have to be made, based on data from the 502 study participants.

In most situations, it is not possible to know the size of the target population, nor is it feasible to evaluate them all. For example, finding the prevalence of adult smokers in the UK would require many millions of adults to complete a survey; and knowing the risk of developing heart disease among females in the US would require a study of every female who ever lived there and knowing her heart disease status. The study population therefore usually represents only a very small proportion of the target population, even though the latter is of ultimate interest.

In the VDP study, 207 out of 502 (41%) participants were classified as a binge drinker, as shown below:

Prevalence of binge drinking

All UK VDPs (n = 767)   ?? (true effect, i.e. true prevalence)
Study of 502 VDPs   41% (observed prevalence)

The best estimate of the true prevalence is 41%, but it would be inappropriate to say that the true value is exactly 41%. If there had been other studies, the observed prevalence could be 45%, 38%, and so on; all different due to natural variation (or chance) and the fact that there just happened to be a few more or a few less reported binge drinkers in each study. The observed prevalence (41%) and the sample size (N = 502) are used to produce a **95% confidence interval (CI)**, which essentially produces a range of values for the true prevalence:

95% CI = observed prevalence ± 1.96 × standard error of the prevalence

1.96 is associated with having a 95% interval (2.5% at the lower and upper ends) and assuming a Normal (or Gaussian) distribution[#]:

$$\text{Standard error} = \sqrt{\frac{(\text{prevalence}) \times (1 - \text{prevalence})}{N}} = \sqrt{\frac{(0.41) \times (1 - 0.41)}{502}} = 0.022$$

Standard error is a measure of the precision of the estimate, given the study size. It indicates how far the observed estimate is expected to be from the true value (a concept established using statistical methodology). Small studies have large standard errors, so the true effect is less certain. In contrast, large studies have small standard errors, and the estimates they produce should be closer to the true value, and therefore be more precise.

$$95\% \text{ CI} = 0.41 \pm 1.96 \times 0.022$$
$$= 0.37 \text{ to } 0.45$$

[#] That is, if we had many estimates of the prevalence, a histogram of their distribution would be symmetric (bell shaped).

Interpretation

The best estimate of the true prevalence is 41%.

But it is not certain that the true value is exactly 41%.

There is 95% certainty that whatever the true value is, it should be between 37 and 45%[#].

(This is quite a narrow range, due to having a large sample size of n = 502.)

[#] Technically, there is 95% certainty that the range 37–45% contains the true value.

Figure 2.3 illustrates the concept of 95% CIs, in which it is assumed that the true prevalence is known (here 40%). There are 20 hypothetical studies, each of the same size (n = 502 VDPs), but including different participants. For each

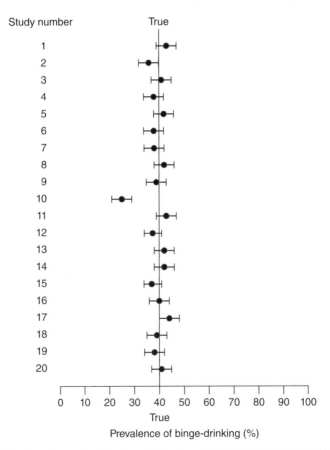

Figure 2.3 Twenty studies, each estimating what the prevalence of binge drinking could be among all dental VDPs, with 95% CIs; 19 are expected to contain the true prevalence, but 1 (5%) is not, by chance alone.

study, there is an estimate of the true value, which may be below, above, or equal to the true value (the variation is due to chance). Because the 95% CIs contain the true value 95% of the time (19 in 20 studies), 1 of the 20 studies is expected to miss it, just by chance (bad luck). Therefore, a study that produces unusual or unexpected findings could simply be the one among 20 studies; the result is not necessarily due to any problem with the design or conduct.

By using 95% CIs, the estimate of the true effect is not restricted to a single number. Small studies tend to have wide intervals, reflecting the high degree of uncertainty inherent in most such studies. Very wide 95% CIs are not useful. Large studies tend to yield more precise results, and because these should be closer to the true values, the CI range should be narrow.

95% CIs can be calculated for any type of summary measure for a single group of participants, and the principle and interpretation are the same as that given earlier:

- Percentage or proportion
- Mean
- Median
- Survival or event rate at a single time point
- Median survival

Some CIs can be calculated manually, while others require statistical software, but they have the same format

95% CI = observed summary measure $\pm 1.96 \times$ standard error of the measure

In the example of the serum cholesterol values on page 28, where the mean was 6.4 mmol/L, the standard error of the mean is 0.248 (standard error = standard deviation/$\sqrt{}$number of people), so the 95% CI is 5.9 to 6.9.

Interpretation

The best estimate of the true mean is 6.4 mmol/L.

It is not entirely certain that it is exactly 6.4 mmol/L.

There is 95% certainty that the true mean should be somewhere between 5.9 and 6.9 mmol/L

2.6 Understanding risk and risk factors

What is risk?

'Counting people' and time-to-event endpoints both produce **risk**. Risk is a common general term used in many observational studies and clinical trials, to describe the effect of an exposure or intervention on a specified disorder, and sometimes only used for an individual. Public health education and clinical practice use measures of risk [4, 5], and compare risks (between exposed and unexposed groups or between those with and without a new intervention), to justify, for example, recommended changes in lifestyle habits or the use of a particular intervention. Risk can be any of the following:

- The chance of having a certain characteristic or of changing a lifestyle habit (e.g. stop smoking)
- The chance of developing a disorder for the first time
- The chance of dying earlier than expected

Chance is taken to be the same as probability, but it has a different meaning here than when considering natural variability (and the concept of statistical significance, see Section 3.3).

The word 'risk' often implies something bad, such as death or occurrence of cancer or heart disease. However, risk can be applied to any type of event, for example, the:

- Chance of surviving 5 years after diagnosis
- Chance of not experiencing severe pain after surgery

Risk can be applied to individuals who do not have the disorder of interest, or to those who have it already. For example,

- Among people who do not have cancer, risk could be:
  - o The chance of developing cancer in a year
  - o The chance of developing cancer over a lifetime
- Among people who already have cancer, risk could be:
  - o The chance of dying
  - o The chance of the cancer coming back (when clinical evidence indicated that it had gone after initial treatment)
  - o The chance of the cancer progressing

Risk is not a single fixed number for a particular individual. It will change as additional relevant information is considered (Figure 2.4). For example, approximately 150,000 people have a stroke each year in the UK, among about 50 million adults aged ≥18 years: a background risk of 0.003 (or 3 in 1000). Either an individual will have a stroke (probability = 1) or they will not (probability = 0), but this will not be known with certainty until the stroke occurs or the person has died from some other cause. As more information, such as age, sex, dietary habits, and smoking status, is incorporated, the risk estimate will move closer to either 0 or 1. Increasing age will move the risk closer to 1; while not being a smoker moves it closer to 0.

It is difficult, if not impossible, to predict with complete certainty what will happen to an individual, so when risk is examined, it is almost always risk relating to a *group* of people. For example, if the risk of having a stroke for a man aged 60 who smokes is 0.007 over a year (7 per 1000), there is no way to tell with certainty what happens to this particular man in relation to stroke. However, it is expected, with some reliability, that in 1000 similar men (all aged 60 and all of whom smoke), 7 would have a stroke and the rest would not. But it is not possible to know who these seven men are until the strokes have occurred.

Two types of outcome measures presented in previous sections (2.2 and 2.4) directly involve estimating risk for a group when summarising data. 'Counting people' endpoints provide the proportion or percentage of participants who have a specified event, and time-to-event data can yield the event rate from a Kaplan–Meier plot. Both are measures of risk. Endpoints based on 'taking measurements on people' (Section 2.3) can also be used to examine risk but <u>only</u> after it has been categorised. For example, if the outcome is blood

A person either will or will not experience the event of interest (over a specified time period or their lifetime)
Until the event is observed (or the person dies from something else), what will happen cannot be predicted with complete certainty

All risk estimates are on a scale that lies between
0 = definitely does not have the disorder of interest, and
1 = definitely does have the disorder of interest

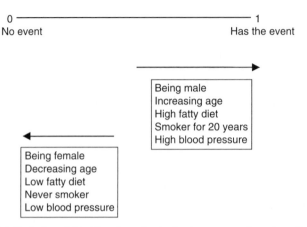

```
0 ──────────────────────────────────────── 1
No event                              Has the event
```

Being male
Increasing age
High fatty diet
Smoker for 20 years
High blood pressure

Being female
Decreasing age
Low fatty diet
Never smoker
Low blood pressure

Figure 2.4 Illustration of risk. There is no fixed value for a person; the value will change according to more information considered. The aforementioned factors relate to the risk of developing stroke, and knowing each of them will increase or decrease the risk value (like a sliding scale).

pressure, the study could examine the risk of developing *high* blood pressure, by first specifying a cut-off: high blood pressure could be defined as systolic blood pressure >140 mmHg and diastolic blood pressure >90 mmHg. It is then possible to consider this as a 'counting people' endpoint (how many do or do not have high blood pressure).

Incidence and prevalence

Two common measures of disease occurrence are **incidence** and **prevalence** (Box 2.2), but they measure quite different aspects. Incidence is the number of *newly diagnosed* cases of a particular disorder, as a proportion of the total number of individuals during a specified time period. Prevalence is a measure of disease status, or other event or characteristic. When referring to disease status, prevalence could include newly diagnosed cases and those who have had the disorder for some time, and so can often be larger than incidence. Prevalence will depend on the incidence and disease duration, and is a measure of the burden of a disorder in a particular population. Both incidence and prevalence are taken to be measures of risk.

For example, there could be 50 new cases of lung cancer among 10,000 smokers over 1 year. Because someone could develop lung cancer at any time during their life, the incidence can either be examined during a specified time

---

Box 2.2 Incidence and prevalence

Incidence: <u>New</u> cases of a specified disorder (or attribute) among a group of people, during a specified time period, for example in 1000 people the:
- number of newly diagnosed cases of thyroid cancer over 12 months
- number of newly diagnosed cases of asthma over a 5-year period
- number of people who start smoking for the first time at age 16

Example: 50 new cases of lung cancer observed in 6000 people who, together, have been observed for 12,000 person-years:

Incidence = 50/12,000 = 0.004, or 4 per 1000 per year

Prevalence: People with the disorder (or attribute) measured at one point in time, for example in 1000 people the:
- number of people currently living with thyroid cancer in 2010
- number of people who have asthma, 2011–2013
- number of people who currently smoke in 2012

These numbers are expressed as a proportion of the number of individuals in a particular population, but there is no time unit.

Example: 100 people who have asthma among 800 randomly selected individuals in 2011:

Prevalence = 100/800 = 0.125, or 12.5% (or 125 per 1000)

Box 2.3 Expressing incidence in relation to person-years rather than number of participants

Observational study of exercise and the risk of colon cancer [6]:

Participants without cancer enrolled in the study 1995–1996

Data collected up to 2003, where possible

Number of men who exercised or played sports ≥5 times per week: 62,688

Men were followed up for an *average* of 6.7 years (420,413/62,688), some more than this, and some less

Number of person-years among these men: 420,413 (~6.7 × 62,688)

Number of men who developed colon cancer for the first time: 431

Incidence: 6.9 per 1000 men (431/62,688) over 6.7 years, or

1.0 per 1000 person years (431/420,413)

Incidence should take account of time

---

period (e.g. 1 year or 5 years) or up to a certain time point, usually over a person's whole lifetime (**cumulative incidence**).

When incidence is expressed as a proportion of the total number of people in the group that has the event of interest, this approach does not allow for people with different lengths of follow-up, which is usually the case in observational studies. It is often more accurate to express incidence as a proportion of the number of **person-years at risk** (Box 2.3). If one subject has been

---

Box 2.4 Characteristics of incidence and prevalence

Incidence rate	Prevalence
Can be difficult to measure if not routinely collected (as part of a registry or prospective study)	Can be easier to measure using retrospective or cross-sectional studies
Suitable for acute disorders (e.g. cancer, stroke, heart attack, and influenza)	Suitable for chronic disorders, from which patients can suffer for many years or which may be lifelong (e.g. asthma, diabetes, and Alzheimer's disease)
Does not depend on survival from the disorder or disease duration	Depends on how well the patient population responds to treatments (e.g. survival) and disease duration
Can be easier to forecast trends over time rather than prevalence	Can be difficult to forecast trends over time because of changes in survival and disease duration

---

followed up (observed) in the study for 2 years and another for 8 years, together, they have provided 10 person-years of follow-up. The length of follow-up for each person is only until they have experienced the event of interest; if the event has not occurred, it is the time until they had the last assessment or contact with the researcher. For example, if the outcome is stroke and a participant suffered one 3 years after entry to the study and then died 2 years later, their follow-up is three person-years, not five. This is because the calculation is based on the length of time **at risk**. Once the subject has had a stroke, the concept of risk for him/her no longer exists.

Prevalence is the number of people who have a certain attribute or disorder, calculated at one point in time or within a specified time period. Unlike incidence, it cannot be represented as a rate. For many attributes, prevalence can be obtained easily, for example, the proportion of people who are current smokers, or the proportion of pregnant women who give birth at home.

However, should a study focussing on the prevalence of breast cancer only include women currently being treated for breast cancer, or should it also include those who had cancer but finished treatment in the previous 6 months? In this instance, prevalence is not so easily defined.

Box 2.4 shows some characteristics of incidence and prevalence.

Comparing incidence or prevalence
Comparing incidence rates (or prevalences) can be useful, for example, when investigating whether the incidence of cancer is different in one geographical location compared with another or whether it changes over time for a single location or comparing the rates between an exposed and unexposed group. However, examining the crude incidence rates could be inappropriate, because

Box 2.5 Standardisation of rates of disease, such as incidence, prevalence, or mortality; with age as the standardisation factor (as either whole years or age categories) [4,5]

Direct standardisation

When comparing incidence between two groups (e.g. two cities, or male/female), a **standardised incidence rate** is produced for each group. It is essentially a weighted average of the observed incidence from each age category in each group being compared, where the weight is the proportion of individuals (or person-years) in each age category from the standard population. It represents total incidence for each group, assuming that they had the same age structure, and expressed as, for example, per 1000 per year, or per 1000 person-years. If comparing prevalence, the result is called **standardised prevalence rate**, and for death rates it is **standardised mortality rate**.

Indirect standardisation

This produces a **standardised incidence ratio (SIR)**, which is the total number of observed cases in a group divided by the expected number (which comes from applying the age-specific incidence in the standard population to person-years in each age category from the group of interest). The SIR will always be 1 in the standard population, <1 indicates that the rate in one group is lower than expected, and >1 that it is higher. Sometimes, the SIR is multiplied by 100. If comparing prevalence, the result is called **standardised prevalence ratio**, and for death rates it is **standardised mortality ratio**.

of differences in age or other factors. There are two methods which can allow for age (or any other factor) (Box 2.5). When comparing measures of risk between groups, one group, or another defined population is identified as the **standard population**, which is used to 'standardise' the rates. These rates can then be compared directly. When comparing over time, e.g. 1995–2010, one year must be made the standard, usually the first year (1995). Standardisation is a long-established approach but regression analyses (Chapter 4) are more often used now in many situations, particularly when examining associations.

Examining incidence or prevalence over time can also be used to forecast what they might be in the future. This is of particular use, for example, to pharmaceutical companies or health service providers, to answer questions such as:

- What budget is needed for when a new drug is licensed, given the expected number of patients that could require it?
- How much could obesity-related illnesses cost a health service over the coming years, given the number of expected cases?

Any projections are guesses, and the further into the future the estimates, the more unreliable they may become. Both incidence and prevalence are influenced by a variety of factors (Figure 2.5), several of which are difficult to

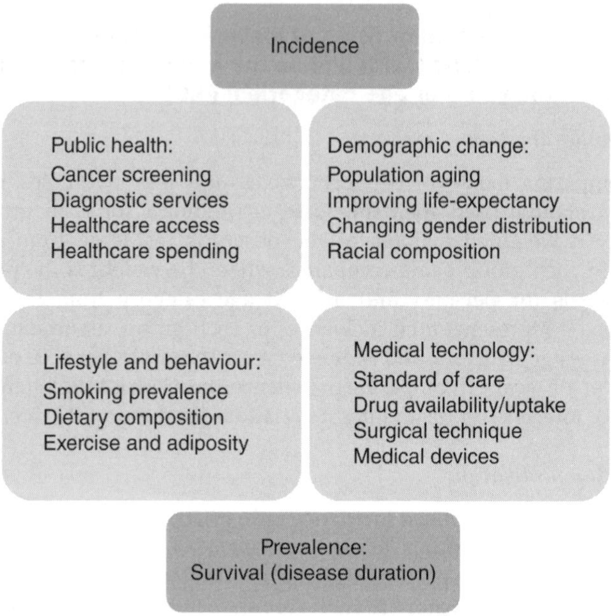

Figure 2.5 Features of a population that can influence incidence and prevalence and therefore how reliably they can be forecasted or predicted (prevalence will also depend on incidence).

incorporate into the modelling associated with forecasting. A clear (increasing or decreasing) trend that has been observed in the past several years may not continue in subsequent years.

2.7 Risk factors and investigating association and causality

A **risk factor** is a characteristic (e.g. lifestyle habit, biological measurement, imaging marker, or genetic factor) that is associated with an *increase* or *decrease* in a person's chance of having or developing a disorder (or early death). Examples are:
- Age
- Smoking
- Blood pressure
- Diet (e.g. eating lots of fruits and vegetables)
- Serum cholesterol
- Breast lesion found on a mammogram
- BRCA 1 gene for breast cancer

Some risk factors could also be investigated in relation to an intermediate outcome, for example, blood pressure is a risk factor for stroke, and could be used to examine how the risk of stroke increases with increasing blood pressure. However, to examine the association between salt intake and blood pressure, salt is the risk factor, and blood pressure is defined as the outcome.

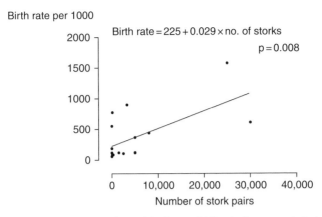

Figure 2.6 Association between storks and the human birth rate (human and stork data for 17 European countries). Source: Matthews, 2000 [7]. Reproduced by permission of John Wiley and Sons Ltd.

It is important to distinguish between association and causality. When examining the effect of a risk factor on a disorder, the association can be casual or non-casual. Many outcomes can be shown to be associated with an exposure, but the interpretation in a biological context is an important step. For example, a study could show that the risk of drowning in a population (the outcome) increases with increasing ice cream sales (the exposure), that is, that drowning and ice cream consumption are associated with each other. Technically, ice cream in this example is a risk factor, but it is unlikely to be a cause of drowning. The two are only associated through the confounder, 'time of year'. As temperature increases, more people swim, therefore more are at risk of drowning. At the same time, more people tend to buy ice cream. There is no direct causal relationship between these two factors.

Figure 2.6 is another example to illustrate this. It is based on the myth once told by parents when asked by children where babies come from (i.e. they answered that storks, a species of bird, delivered babies to the home). There is clearly an association between the number of stork pairs and the human birth rate (storks could arguably be referred to as a risk factor), but there is no real (causal) link. 'Cause' should mean that the exposure and the outcome are biologically linked in some way, though we may or may not know the actual mechanism.

Many observational studies can only examine association but may be reported in journals or the media to give the impression of a causal link.

Investigating causality

In its purest form, the statement 'an exposure X *causes* outcome Y' means that everyone who has X always gets Y, and those who do not have X never get Y. While such firm relationships exist in sciences such as chemistry and physics, they are hardly ever seen in studies of human health. For example, one of the strongest risk factors for lung cancer is being a lifelong smoker. However, not

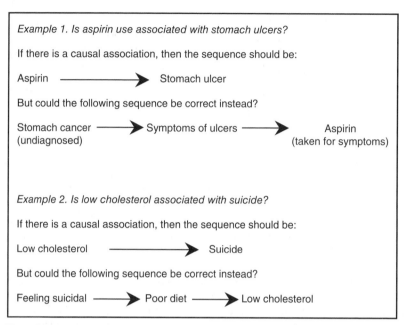

Example 1. Is aspirin use associated with stomach ulcers?

If there is a causal association, then the sequence should be:

Aspirin ───────────▶ Stomach ulcer

But could the following sequence be correct instead?

Stomach cancer ────▶ Symptoms of ulcers ────▶ Aspirin
(undiagnosed)   (taken for symptoms)

Example 2. Is low cholesterol associated with suicide?

If there is a causal association, then the sequence should be:

Low cholesterol ──────────▶ Suicide

But could the following sequence be correct instead?

Feeling suicidal ────▶ Poor diet ────▶ Low cholesterol

Figure 2.7 How time sequence is important in determining causality.

all smokers develop lung cancer, and some never-smokers do. There are other exposures, such as asbestos, that can also lead to lung cancer. Because most disorders have multiple causes, and many exposures can lead to several disorders, it is difficult to establish a causal link between a risk factor (exposure) and an outcome measure in the same way that other sciences can. However, in order to change public health education or clinical practice, it is important to be able to make some conclusions (inferences) about causality. In reports of observational trials, the statement 'X causes Y' really means that 'X is a cause of Y', and that the researchers believe they have accumulated sufficient evidence to conclude a causal relationship.

Associations can be found between many exposures and outcomes in studies of human health (illustrated in the two examples above), but it is a big 'step up' to claim that an association represents a causal link. In order to call (or 'upgrade') a potential risk factor a causal factor, several pieces of evidence are required. 'Criteria' for causality have been suggested in the past; the most well-known being those by Bradford Hill [8], with others based on this [9]. However, 'criteria' implies a checklist of items that require all are met before concluding the presence of a causal relationship with almost complete certainty. This is usually difficult to do. Box 2.6 shows the main *features* of causality. No feature, individually, can provide evidence for a causal link, but the more that are met reliably, the more evidence exists to make a conclusion about causality. Establishing time sequence is fundamental (Figure 2.7). For example, in considering whether aspirin could be a cause of stomach ulcers, the

---

Box 2.6 Features of causality

• The exposure must come before the outcome (time sequence)
• The association between the exposure (risk factor) and outcome should be clinically important, and statistically significant, after allowing for confounders and bias
• Risk of having the outcome should increase or decrease with increasing levels of the exposure (dose–response)
• The risk should decrease if the exposure is removed (reversibility)
• There should be consistency in results between independent studies, including between people with different characteristics
• There should be biological plausibility for a causal link (could come from experimental/laboratory studies)

---

prevalence of those with ulcers could be higher in aspirin users than non-users, providing initial evidence of an association. However, people with ulcers may have symptoms for which they then take aspirin; aspirin use would therefore not be a cause, but rather a consequence of having the disorder. A similar explanation could be made for low cholesterol and attempted suicide.

The existence of a strong association is often specified as a requirement for causality, implying that such an association is more likely to be causal. However, there are many causal relationships where the association is moderate or relatively weak (e.g. passive smoking and lung cancer, among never-smokers). The totality of the evidence must be considered (Box 2.6).

One feature missing from Box 2.6 is

2.8 Key points

• Researchers should have clearly defined outcome measures (endpoints).
• Outcome measures can only be one of three types: 'counting people', 'taking measurements on people', or time-to-event data.
• Determining the category of outcome measure is essential to study design and analysis and interpretation of the findings.
• Data from all three categories can be summarised using a single number.
• Data can be shown in a diagram using bar charts ('counting people'), scatter plots ('taking measurements on people'), or Kaplan–Meier curves (time-to-event).
• Uncertainty over the true value of the summary number is addressed by using a 95% CI.
• Risk (chance) is associated with having or developing a well-defined event, and for an individual will change as more useful information is known on them.
• Incidence and prevalence are two common measures of risk.
• It is often easy to find an association between an exposure (e.g. risk factor) and an outcome (disorder).
• But making conclusions about causality requires much evidence, of which association is only one feature.

References

1. Kirkwood BR, Sterne JAC. *Essential Medical Statistics*. Blackwell Science. Second Edition (2003).
2. Petrie A, Sabin C. *Medical Statistics at a Glance*. Wiley-Blackwell. Third Edition (2009).
3. Bland JM. *An Introduction to Medical Statistics*. Oxford University Press. Third Edition (2000).
4. Rothman KJ. *Epidemiology: An Introduction*. Oxford University Press. First Edition (2002).
5. Silman AJ, Macfarlane GJ. *Epidemiological Studies: A Practical Guide*. Cambridge University Press. Second Edition (2002).
6. Howard RA, Freedman DM, Park Y, Hollenbeck A, Schatzkin A, Leitzmann MF. Physical activity, sedentary behavior, and the risk of colon and rectal cancer in the NIH-AARP Diet and Health Study. *Cancer Causes Control* 2008;19(9):939–53.
7. Matthews R. Storks deliver babies (p=0.008). *Teach Stat* 2000;22(2):36–8.
8. Hill AB. The environment and disease: association or causation? *Proc R Soc Med* 1965;58:295–300.
9. Wald NJ. *Epidemiological Approach* An Approach to Epidemology in Medicine (4th Edition), Woltson Institute of Preventive Medicine, Royal Society of Medicine (2004).

CHAPTER 3

Effect sizes

Before presenting types of observational studies (Chapter 5–8), it is worth knowing how they are analyzed. Examining the effect of an exposure (including risk factors) on an outcome measure should be performed in a way that can be quantified and communicated to others. This chapter covers the main ways of achieving this using **effect sizes**. Chapter 4 introduces regression analyses which are common statistical methods that produce effect sizes.

3.1 Effect sizes

Sections 2.1–2.4 covered the main methods of summarising data from several study participants when describing a *single* group of people. However, most observational studies compare two or more groups, or examine the relationship between two factors.

An **effect size** is a single quantitative summary measure used to interpret data from observational studies and clinical trials. It is often obtained by comparing the outcome measure between two groups. The choice of effect size depends on the type of outcome measure used: 'counting people' (binary/categorical data), 'taking measurements on people' (continuous data), or time-to-event data. The most common effects sizes are summarised in Box 3.1, and each is covered in the sections below. They can be used for measures of risk (incidence, prevalence, and mortality rates), or the average (mean or median) of a measurement.

Before performing even simple analyses of effect sizes, it is always useful to examine the data using plots (diagrams). By graphically showing the data, such as scatter plots or bar charts, it is possible to see the extent of variability and potential outliers, or to examine how the cumulative risk changes over time, as with Kaplan–Meier survival curves. Relatively few published reports of observational studies present diagrams.

'Counting people' outcome measures

Box 3.2 is an example of a survey of newly qualified dental undergraduates [1]. Each percentage (or proportion) indicates the **risk** (or **chance**). In this example, the risk (which can also be called **prevalence**) of hazardous alcohol consumption among males is 6.7%, and for females it is 1.8%. It is clear that

A Concise Guide to Observational Studies in Healthcare, First Edition. Allan Hackshaw.
© 2015 John Wiley & Sons, Ltd. Published 2015 by John Wiley & Sons, Ltd.

Box 3.1 Effect sizes obtained by comparing two groups of study participants (e.g. exposed and unexposed)

Type of outcome measure	Summary measure in each group*	Effect size obtained by comparing two groups	How do we estimate the true effect?
'Counting people' (categorical data)	Percentage (proportion)	Relative risk (risk ratio) Risk difference (attributable risk)	95% CI
	Odds	Odds ratio	95% CI
'Taking measurements on people' (continuous data)	Mean (and standard deviation)	Difference between two means (mean difference)	95% CI
	Median (and interquartile range)	Difference between two medians	95% CI
Time-to-event	Kaplan–Meier curve Event rate at a specific time point	Hazard ratio Risk difference	95% CI 95% CI

CI, confidence interval (other CIs can be used instead, e.g. 90 or 99%).
*see Chapter 2.

---

more males were heavy drinkers than females, but this needs to be quantified using a single number.

The effect size for this type of outcome measure is either the ratio (called **relative risk** or **risk ratio**) or the difference (called **absolute risk difference**) between the two risks:

1. Relative risk = 6.7/1.8% = 3.7: Males were 3.7 times more likely to engage in hazardous consumption than females.
2. Risk difference = 6.7–1.8% = +4.9 percentage points[#]: Among 100 males, there were 4.9 *more* heavy drinkers than in a group of 100 females. (The plus sign indicates there would be *more* events; a minus sign indicates *fewer* events.) This effect size can also be called **attributable risk**, because it measures the absolute risk that is due to the exposure (in this example heavy alcohol use).

The **comparison** or **reference group**, chosen by the researcher, must always be made clear. It is insufficient to say that 'Males are 3.7 times more likely to be heavy drinkers' but correct to assert that 'Males are 3.7 times more likely to be heavy drinkers *compared with females*'. If the reference group were males, the relative risk would be 0.3 (1.8/6.7%): females are 0.3 times as likely to engage in hazardous consumption as males.

[#] **Percentage points** is preferable to %, because the latter can be confused with percentage change in risk (presented later in this section), but they have different interpretations.

Box 3.2 Example of a study where the outcome measure is based on 'counting people' (binary/categorical data) [1]

Study participants: 502 newly qualified dental undergraduates vocational dental practitioners (VDPs), who responded out of a total of 767.

Objective: Are male VDPs more or less likely than females to have hazardous alcohol consumption?

Location: All VDPs on the national register in the UK in 2005.

Exposure: Gender (male or female).

Outcome measure: Hazardous alcohol consumption (heavy drinking) in the previous week defined as ≥50 units per week for males and ≥36 units for females.

Results	Males	Females
No. of participants	224	278
No. heavy drinkers	15	5
Percentage (risk)	6.7% (15/224)	1.8% (5/278)
Relative risk (males vs. females)	3.7 (6.7/1.8%)	
Absolute risk difference	+4.9 percentage points (6.7–1.8%)	

The *no effect* value

If there were no difference in alcohol drinking habits between the two groups, each would have the same risk of hazardous consumption. The relative risk (the ratio of the two risks) would be one, and the risk difference would be zero. These are called the **no effect values**, and they are used when interpreting confidence intervals and p-values (Sections 3.2 and 3.3).

Direction of the effect

Relative risk and absolute risk difference indicate the magnitude of the effect, but not the direction, that is, whether the outcome in one group is better or worse than another. This will depend on what is being measured (Box 3.3).

Converting relative risk to percentage change in risk

Relative risks of 0.5 or 2.0 are easy to interpret; the risk is half or twice as large as in the reference group. However, values of 0.85 or 1.30 are less intuitive; the risks are 0.85 or 1.30 times as large as that in the reference group. Converting relative risk to a **percentage change in risk** is an attempt to make it more interpretable (Box 3.4).

Relative effects (relative risk) or absolute effects (risk difference)?

Relative risk (risk ratio) and risk difference each provide different information about the study results. Relative risks tend to be similar across different populations, indicating the effect of an exposure *generally*. They do not usually depend on the underlying rate of disease. A relative risk of 0.5 means that the risk is halved from whatever it is in a particular population, for example,

---

Box 3.3 Interpreting the direction of an effect depends on whether the outcome measure is a 'good' or 'bad' thing

	Example*	Group A (%)	Group B (%)	Relative risk	Risk difference	Comment
'Bad' outcome measure	Risk of dying	10	7	1.43	+3 percentage points	Group A has a *worse* outcome than B
	Risk of experiencing pain					
'Good' outcome measure	Risk of stopping smoking	15	10	1.50	−5 percentage points	Group A has a *better* outcome than B
	Risk of being alive					

*The word **chance** could be used instead of **risk**.

Box 3.4 Converting a relative risk (risk ratio) to percentage change in risk (generally done for values <2.0)

Relative risk (RR)	How far is it from the no effect value (1.0)? (RR − 1)	Multiply by 100 to get percentage change (RR − 1) × 100	
0.75	−0.25	−25%	Relative risk reduction (or risk reduction)
1.38	+0.38	+38%	Excess relative risk (or excess risk)

Positive sign: the risk is increased compared with the reference group.
Negative sign: the risk is decreased.

---

a background incidence of 1 per 1000 reducing to 0.5 per 1000, or 20 per 1000 reducing to 10 per 1000. However, risk difference reflects (depends on) the underlying rate, and so will vary between populations. It indicates the effect *in a particular population*, that is, a measure of impact.

As a disorder becomes more common, relative risk is not expected to change much, but risk difference will increase. An exposure has a greater impact on a population when the disorder is common. Table 3.1 illustrates this. Smoking is the *strongest* risk factor for those with the largest relative risks that is, lung cancer (14.6) and chronic obstructive pulmonary disease (COPD) (14.2), while there is only a moderate association between smoking and ischaemic heart disease (relative risk 1.62). However, the number of *extra* deaths among

Table 3.1 Relative risk and absolute risk difference for disorders that have varying underlying death rates, using an observational study of smoking [2].

Outcome measure	Annual death rate per 100,000 men		Relative risk	Absolute risk difference (per 100,000)*
	Current smokers (any tobacco)	Never-smokers		
	a	b	a / b	a − b
Lung cancer	249	17	14.6	+232
Head and neck cancer	60	9	6.7	+51
Ischaemic heart disease	1001	619	1.62	+382
COPD	156	11	14.2	+145

*The number of extra deaths among 100,000 smokers, compared with 100,000 never-smokers.

100,000 smokers is 232 and 145 for lung and COPD, respectively, both of which are lower than the number of extra deaths due to heart disease, 382. Even though the relationship (relative risk) between smoking and heart disease is much weaker than for lung cancer, the impact on public health is greater, because heart disease is more common. Similarly, although there is a strong association for head and neck cancer (relative risk 6.7), there are only 51 extra cases per 100,000 smokers.

Because risk difference varies between populations, relative risk is the most commonly reported effect size. Risk difference should be examined in addition to relative risk when evaluating the impact on a population.

Relative risk or odds ratio?

An **odds ratio** is sometimes reported instead of relative risk. It has useful mathematical properties used by many statistical methods, especially the regression methods (Chapter 4). **Risk** and **odds** are different ways of presenting the likelihood of having a disorder (or other event):

Risk: $1/n$, e.g. $1/10$

Odds: $1/n–1$, e.g. $1/9$

The denominator for risk is all individuals, but for odds it is only unaffected individuals.

Table 3.2 illustrates odds ratio and relative risk, for different prevalence. In Table 3.2B, it would be incorrect to interpret the odds ratio of 14.8 as a 14-fold increase in risk (or 138% excess risk). The risk has been increased 2.5 fold (or 150%), indicated by the relative risk, but the odds in males are 14.8 times greater than the odds in females.

Odds ratio is the effect size calculated from case–control studies; cohort studies can be used to produce either an odds ratio or relative risk.

How big is the effect?

When interpreting relative risks or odds ratios, it is useful to judge whether the effect is small, moderate, or large. Although this can be a subjective exercise, it considers the importance of the association between an exposure and outcome measure in context. Figure 3.1 is an approximate classification.

Table 3.2 Calculation of relative risk and odds ratio using the survey of VDPs (newly qualified dental graduates) (from Box 3.2), and how they can be similar (disorder is uncommon) or very different (disorder is common, >20%).

	Males	*Females*
(A) Prevalence of heavy drinking is relatively uncommon		
Heavy drinker	15 (a)	5 (b)
Not heavy drinker	209 (c)	273 (d)
Total	224	278

Relative risk of being a heavy drinker = (15/224) ÷ (5/278) = 3.7

Odds of being a heavy drinker among males = 15/209 (a/b)
Odds of being a heavy drinker among females = 5/273 (c/d)
Odds ratio is (15/209) ÷ (5/273) = (a × d)/(b × c) = 3.9

Relative risk and odds ratio are similar

(B) Prevalence of heavy drinking is common (hypothetical results)

	Males	*Females*
Heavy drinker	200 (a)	100 (b)
Not heavy drinker	24 (c)	178 (d)
Total	224	278

Relative risk of being a heavy drinker = (200/224) ÷ (100/278) = 2.5
Odds ratio of being a heavy drinker = (200/24) ÷ (100/178) = 14.8
[same calculation as the cross-product (200 × 178)/(24 × 100)]

Relative risk and odds ratio are very different

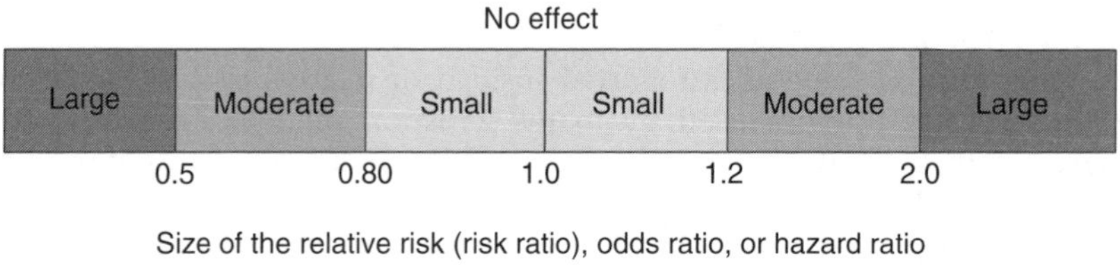

No effect

Large	Moderate	Small	Small	Moderate	Large

0.5   0.80   1.0   1.2   2.0

Size of the relative risk (risk ratio), odds ratio, or hazard ratio

Example	Approximate relative risk (RR) of developing lung cancer	Strength of association
Active life-long smoker (compared with never-smokers)	RR = 20	Very strong
Passive smoking (exposed compared with unexposed never smokers)	RR = 1.30	Moderate (possibly small)
Women drinking 3 or 4 units of alcohol per day (compared with non-drinkers)	RR = 1.15	Fairly weak

Figure 3.1 Approximate guide to judging whether relative effect sizes are associated with small, moderate, or large effects.

Table 3.3 Illustration of relative versus absolute effects.

Risk of an event		Relative risk	Risk difference
Exposed	*Unexposed*		
3 per 100	1 per 100	3	2 per 100
3 per 1,000,000	1 per 1,000,000	3	2 per 1,000,000

Using *relative effects* can make the association between an exposure and outcome appear more important than it really is. An extreme example is shown in Table 3.3. The relative risk is 3 in both cases, representing a trebling of risk (or a 200% increase in risk) which is considered large, but the *absolute risk difference* in the second row of the table actually represents only two additional persons with the disorder among every one million exposed. This is a negligible effect, in terms of impact on a population. The classification of effects as small to large should therefore be applied separately to relative risk or absolute risk difference, and it may not be the same.

The effect size should be examined after adjusting for the effects of potential confounders (using regression methods in Chapter 4) otherwise conclusions on the relationship, especially if causality is inferred, could be questionable. Very large effects (e.g. a relative risk of 10 or more) are unlikely to be completely explained by confounding and bias, so if important confounding and bias have been ignored the conclusion probably remains the same, but there might be uncertainty over the size of the effect (the relative risk could be 5 instead of 10 after allowance for confounders, but 5 is still large). Small effects (e.g. relative risk 1.10) could be due to confounding or bias, so more care is needed when interpreting these.

Attributable fraction (or risk)
The risk in the exposed and unexposed groups can be used to calculate an **attributable fraction**, of which there are two forms (Box 3.5). Both assume that there is no significant bias or confounding; if there were, the estimates are likely to be lower. Attributable fractions can be used in addition to effect sizes when describing the impact of an exposure (risk factor) on a disorder in a population.

'Taking measurements on people' outcome measures
When using 'taking measurements on people', data are often summarised by the mean and standard deviation, as measures of average and spread (Chapter 2). An appropriate effect size is the **difference between two means** (or **mean difference**). It often has a Normal (Gaussian) distribution, allowing the application of several methods of statistical analyses, including some simple ones. Taking the ratio of two means has an intuitive appeal (in a similar way to the ratio of two risks), but the distribution of ratios is not usually Gaussian, and therefore standard statistical methods often cannot be applied.

If the measurement if obviously non-Gaussian (that is skewed), even after suitable transformations, an effect size could be the difference between two medians.

Box 3.5 Calculating and interpreting attributable fractions (or risk)

$$\text{Attributable fraction (or risk)} = 1 - \frac{1}{\text{Relative risk}}$$

Using Table 3.1, the attributable fraction for lung cancer is 93% $(1-1/14.6)$, and for ischaemic heart disease, it is 38% $(1-1/1.62)$:

Among smokers, the proportion of lung cancer cases due to smoking is 90%.
Among smokers, the proportion of ischaemic heart disease cases due to smoking is 38%.

$$\text{Population attributable fraction}\,(\text{PAF})\,(\text{or risk}) = \frac{P_E(\text{relative risk} - 1)}{1 + P_E(\text{relative risk} - 1)}$$

P_E is the proportion of the population that is exposed.

We assume that 25% of individuals are smokers. The PAF is:
Lung cancer: 77%
Ischaemic heart disease: 13%

77% of all cases of lung cancer in the population are due to smoking.
13% of all cases of ischaemic heart disease in the population are due to smoking.

Consider a study comparing head circumference between men with (57.46 cm) and without (58.04 cm) Alzheimer's disease (see Box 6.3) [3]. The effect size (mean difference) would be $57.46 - 58.04 = -0.58$ cm. This means that males with Alzheimer's disease had a head circumference that was, on average, 0.58 cm *smaller* than unaffected males. Some individuals with Alzheimer's had a head circumference greater than those who were unaffected, some smaller, and others the same size, but *on average* the circumference was smaller. The mean difference, like any other summary measure, is not perfect, in that it cannot represent everyone in the study. The purpose of the effect size is to summarise the endpoint (here head circumference) for a group of people, not for an individual. The standard deviation of the mean difference of 0.18 indicates that the *difference* between the two groups is expected to vary by, on average, 0.18 cm from the mean of −0.58 cm.

How big is the effect?
As with relative risks and odds ratios, it is useful to judge whether a mean difference is clinically important, that is, small, moderate, or large. While this will be obvious in many situations, for several outcome measures based on 'taking measurements on people', this assessment can be made only after considering the original measurement scale:
- In the example of Alzheimer's disease, the mean difference among males was −0.58 cm (5.8 mm). This is a small effect in relation to an average head circumference of about 60 cm.

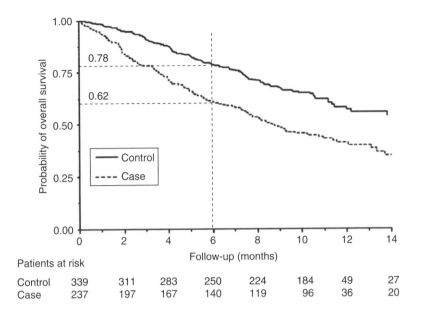

Patients at risk

Control	339	311	283	250	224	184	49	27
Case	237	197	167	140	119	96	36	20

Study participants: 237 cancer patients with known venous thromboembolism (VTE) and 339 cancer patients without VTE
Objective: Is VTE among cancer patients associated with the chance of dying?
Exposure: Presence or absence of VTE
Outcome measure: Overall survival (an event is death from any cause)

Figure 3.2 Kaplan–Meier curves for comparing cancer patients with and without venous thromboembolism (cases and controls, respectively). Source: Agnelli et al 2013 [4]. Reproduced by permission of Springer Science + Business Media.

- If a study endpoint is body weight, and the exposure is a new diet, a weight loss, for example, of 5 kg would probably be interpreted as a moderate effect, while a loss of 0.2 kg would be considered small, but it is also worth considering the starting weight of the person, because a 5 kg loss for someone who initially weighed 55 kg is relatively greater than the same loss in someone who started at 120 kg.

Time-to-event outcome measures
Comparing two groups is presented graphically using two Kaplan–Meier curves (Figure 3.2). The two rows at the bottom of the graph are important, they show the number of **participants at risk** in each group. All participants are alive (event-free) at the start of the study, and the number at risk should equal the total number of individuals in the study (339 + 237). The number of participants at risk, therefore, indicates the reliability of the curves at each time point.

A **hazard ratio** is an effect size in which the risk of an event in one group is compared with the risk in another, at the same time point (obtained by comparing the whole curves). It is interpreted in the same way as relative risk (Box 3.3), and can also be converted to a percentage change in risk (Box 3.4). In the example (Figure 3.2), the hazard ratio is 1.79: the risk of dying is increased by 79% in the cases compared with the controls. If the hazard ratio were 0.60, the risk of dying would be reduced by 40%.

If the outcome measure has an **exponential distribution** (a constant event rate over time), the ratio of the two medians should be close to the hazard ratio. In Figure 3.2, the median survival time is 8.7 months for cases (M1) and 14.3 months for controls (M2). The ratio (M2/M1) is 1.64 (14.3/8.7), which is reasonably close to the observed hazard ratio of 1.79.*

It is also possible to calculate an **absolute risk difference** at a specific time point. For example, the approximate survival rate at 6 months for cases is 62%, and for controls, it is 78% (Figure 3.2), a difference of −16 percentage points. This means that at 6 months, there were 16 *fewer* patients alive among 100 cases compared with 100 controls. An alternative is to use the event (death) rate, which is simply 100 minus the survival rate: cases 38% minus controls 22%, which is a difference of +16 percentage points; an *extra* 16 deaths per 100 cases. Researchers should pre-specify the time point to avoid selecting one that appears to show the largest difference.

A hazard ratio assumes that the effect of an exposure is similar over time, that is, if there is a 25% reduction at 1 year, there should be a similar reduction at 5 years (referred to as an **assumption of proportional hazards**). This assumption clearly does not hold for every time point along the curves, particularly at the very start and at the end, when the curves may come closer together. The hazard ratio thus represents an average effect for most of the time period.

A hazard ratio is not appropriate when the curves cross each other. In Figure 3.3, the hazard ratio is 0.84, but there cannot be a 16% reduction in risk at most time points, because the survival rate is lower in the exposed group at 5 months but slightly higher at 10 months. Here, it is best to report the risk difference at a pre-specified time point as well as the hazard ratio, even though the latter may not be accurate.# Alternatively, it may be possible to obtain the **restricted mean survival time (RMST)** [5] up to a specified time point for each curve, towards the end of follow-up (for the participant with the longest time). This is the mean survival time in each group (the area under the whole curve up to the time point), and the difference between the two areas is the effect size: a difference in mean survival times (Figure 3.3).

Hazard ratio (time-to-event outcomes) and relative risk/odds ratio ('counting people' outcomes) can be interpreted in the same way. Both measure risk, and the main difference is that relative risk or odds ratios ignore the time taken

---

* If the hazard ratio is for exposed versus unexposed (or cases vs. controls), the corresponding ratio of the medians should be unexposed/exposed (or controls/cases).
# Hazard ratios would be provided for completeness because most researchers are used to seeing them.

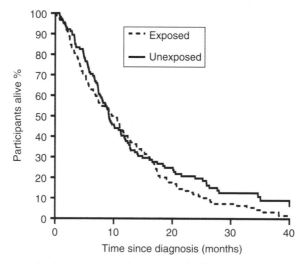

Figure 3.3 An example of survival curves that cross each other, so that the hazard ratio is unlikely to be an appropriate effect size. The hazard ratio is 0.84. The RMST up to 40 months is 13.6 months among the unexposed group and 11.9 months in the exposed group: a mean difference of +1.7 months, indicating that the unexposed group had a mean survival time 1.7 months longer than the exposed group.

for the event to occur, while hazard ratio takes time into account. Interpreting risk difference for these two types of outcome measures is also the same.

3.2 What could the true effect be, given that the study was conducted on a sample of people?

The concept of a 95% CI and estimating a true proportion, mean, or survival time for a single group of individuals was presented in Section 2.5. The same principle is used for effect sizes. The objective is to make conclusions about the target population, even though the study has been conducted on only a small proportion of it.

In the example in Box 3.2, if every VDP responded to the survey, the results would yield the true prevalence of these habits among males and females in the year the study was conducted, and therefore, the true relative risk of hazardous drinking would be known; there is no uncertainty. However, given that 502 out of 767 VDPs responded, a 95% CI is useful, though it assumes that the 265 non-responders have similar characteristics to the responders, which may not be the case.

A **standard error** attempts to quantify by how much the observed effect size differs from the true effect size (similar principle to Section 2.5).[#] The standard

---

[#] It may be difficult to comprehend how the distance between the observed effect and the true effect can be quantified, when the latter is unknown. Established statistical methods have shown that this can be done.

Box 3.6 General definition of a 95% confidence interval (CI)

95% CI for an effect size (e.g. relative risk, odds ratio, hazard ratio, risk difference, or mean difference):

A range within which the **true** effect size is expected to lie, with a high degree of certainty.

If CIs were calculated from many different studies of the same size, 95% of them should contain the true value, and 5% would not.*

$$95\% \text{ CI} = \text{effect size} \pm 1.96 \times \text{standard error}$$

[standard error is calculated on a $\log_e$ scale for relative risk, odds ratio, and hazard ratio]

*The same principle as shown in Figure 2.6.

---

error is then used to calculate a 95% CI (Box 3.6). The formulae are more complex than for a single group and software is more reliable than doing the calculations by hand.

Box 3.7 shows the standard errors and 95% CIs using the results from Box 3.2. The true relative risk is expected to lie somewhere between 1.37 and 10.09, with 95% certainty, so a conservative estimate of the effect is 1.37 (moderate: 37% increase in risk), and an upper estimate is 10.09 (large: 10-fold increase). The interval excludes the no effect value, so the true relative risk is unlikely to be 1.0. There is likely to be a real effect. The 95% CI for a risk difference can also be interpreted in a similar way, except the no effect value is 0.

There is likely to be a real association if the:

95% CI for the relative risk, odds ratio, or hazard ratio excludes the no effect value of 1.

95% CI for the excess risk or risk reduction excludes the no effect value of 0.

95% CI for the risk difference or mean difference excludes the no effect value of 0.

The width of a 95% CI is determined by the size of the standard error, which is influenced by two items, depending on the type of outcome measure (Box 3.8). The most reliable conclusions of a study come from those associated with narrow intervals (Figure 3.4).

It is a common misconception, when describing a CI, that the true effect size lies anywhere within the range with the *same* likelihood. The true value is more likely to lie around the middle of the interval, close to the point estimate used to derive the interval, than at either extreme end. This is an important consideration when the interval just overlaps the no effect value.

Box 3.7 Standard error and 95% CIs for male and female VDPs and the risk of hazardous alcohol drinking (see Box 3.2)

Hazardous alcohol drinking habits

Males   Females
6.7% (15/224)   1.8% (5/278)
a/N_1 b/N_2

		Standard error	95% CI
Relative risk	3.72	0.509	1.37 to 10.09
Odds ratio	3.92	0.524	1.40 to 10.95
Risk difference	+4.9 percentage points	1.84	+1.3 to +8.5

When comparing $P_1 = a/N_1$ versus $P_2 = b/N_2$:

$$\text{Standard error of loge relative risk} = \sqrt{\left[\frac{1}{a} + \frac{1}{b} - \frac{1}{N_1} - \frac{1}{N_2}\right]}$$

$$\text{Standard error of loge odds ratio} = \sqrt{\left[\frac{1}{a} + \frac{1}{b} + \frac{1}{N_1 - a} + \frac{1}{N_2 - b}\right]}$$

$$\text{Standard error of risk difference} = \sqrt{\left[\frac{P_1 \times (1 - P_1)}{N_1} + \frac{P_2 \times (1 - P_2)}{N_2}\right]}$$

Box 3.8 The size of a standard error of an effect size depends on two numbers for each type of outcome measure

Type of outcome measure	Study size	Number of events	Standard deviation
'Counting people' (binary or categorical)	√	√	
'Taking measurements on people' (continuous)	√		√
Time-to-event	√	√	

Small standard errors are produced by large studies, large number of events, or small standard deviations.

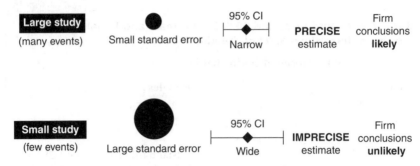

Figure 3.4 How study size affects conclusions.

If interpreting a hazard ratio of 0.85 and 95% CI of 0.65–1.05, most of the range is below the no effect value (indicating benefit). Although the possibility of 'no effect' cannot be excluded reliably, because the interval just includes 1.0, the true hazard ratio is more likely to lie around 0.85 than 1.0 [6]. There is a 50% chance that the interval 0.77 to 0.90 contains the true effect. An association should not be dismissed completely with this kind of result. There is indeed some evidence of an effect from the point estimate, which is always the best guess of the true effect size. In this situation it would be appropriate to assert that 'there is a *suggestion* of an association'.

3.3 Could the observed result be a chance finding in this particular study?

The observed relative risk associated with heavy alcohol drinking (males vs. females) in the VDPs study was 3.72 among the 502 study participants who responded (Box 3.2). What the study is attempting to determine is the effect in all VDPs in 2005, the same concept considered when interpreting 95% CIs. If the study had included *every* VDP, could the true relative risk really be as large as 3.72, or even greater? A more fundamental question is could there, in fact, be no difference at all, and the observed relative risk of 3.72 was just a chance finding in this one particular study, due to natural variation?[#]

In all medical research, the answer to the last question is always '**yes**', and we determine the likelihood of this by calculating a **p-value**. The size of a p-value depends on the difference between the two risks (effect size), the sample size on which each risk is based, and the number of events (i.e. heavy drinkers) (see Figure 3.5).

The p-value for the relative risk of 3.72 is 0.01, where each risk is based on 15/224 and 5/278. If there really were no effect (i.e. males were no more or less likely to be heavy drinkers than females, so the true relative risk was 1.0), a

---

[#] Or if many other studies were conducted, each with 502 subjects, would a relative risk as large as 3.72, or greater, be observed in many of them, assuming there was no real difference in heavy drinking prevalence between males and females?

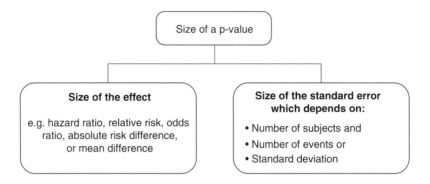

- p-values get smaller with large treatment effects or small standard errors (seen with large studies, many events, or small standard deviations).
- p-values get larger with small treatment effects or large standard errors (seen with small studies, few events, or large standard deviations).

Figure 3.5 Two factors each influence the size of a p-value separately.

value of 3.72 could indeed be seen in some studies, just by chance alone. The p-value of 0.01 indicates that a relative risk as large as 3.72 or greater is expected to occur in only 1 in 100 studies of the same size by chance alone, <u>assuming</u> that there really were no effect. It is therefore *unlikely* (but not impossible) that the observed effect size arose by chance, and so *likely* to reflect a real effect.

The p-value of 0.01 is **two-tailed**. A relative risk of 3.72 or higher (more male drinkers than females), or 1/3.72 (0.27) or lower (fewer male drinkers than females), were both plausible before the study results were known. Any departure from the no effect value is allowed for, in either direction. The p-value is twice as large as a **one-tailed** p-value, which is based on looking only in a single direction (e.g. only more male drinkers than females). Two-tailed p-values are therefore the most conservative, and the most commonly reported, unless there is a clear justification for using a one-tailed value.

All p-values lie on a scale between 1 (definitely no effect) and 0 (definitely an effect) (Figure 3.6). A cut-off of 0.05 is generally accepted to be low enough to guide decision-making, but there is nothing scientific about this level. P-values measure error: the chance of concluding that an association exists, when it does not really. But;

- A p-value ≥ 0.05 does not mean with certainty that there is no effect.
- A p-value < 0.05 does not guarantee there is a real effect.

A p-value can be calculated for any effect size. Because the size of a p-value is influenced by two pieces of information separately (Figure 3.5), it is possible to find:

- Small effect sizes that are not clinically important, with small p-values, when the study is very large or has many events
- Moderate/large effect sizes that have p-values that are > 0.05, when the study is not large enough or has too few events

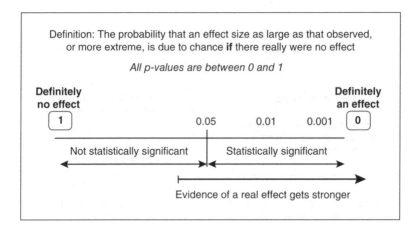

- In general, p-values should be reported to two or three decimal places, unless very small, in which case <0.001 will usually be sufficient.
- Using notation such as 'p < 0.05', 'p > 0.05', or 'not statistically significant' is unacceptable, because it does not distinguish p = 0.04 from p = 0.001 or p = 0.68 from p = 0.06; they each provide very different strengths of evidence.

Figure 3.6 Definition of p-values.

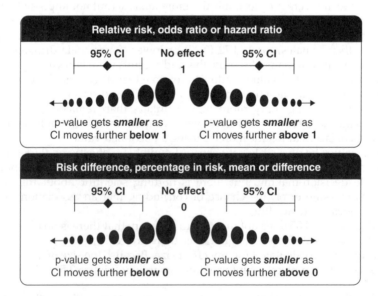

Figure 3.7 Relationship between CIs and p-values where the distance from the effect size to the no effect value is measured in terms of standard errors. If the 95% CI excludes the appropriate no effect value then p-value should be <0.05.

It is difficult to interpret borderline p-values that are just either side of 0.05, particularly those just above 0.05 [6]. Researchers are often unduly influenced by the p-value when interpreting study results. They should focus more on the magnitude of the effect size, its clinical importance, and 95% CI. There is little numerical difference between p=0.045 and p=0.055, yet because of the generally applied cut-off of 0.05, 'an effect' is often concluded for the first p-value and 'no effect' for the second. This is incorrect. There are three possible reasons why a p-value would be ≥0.05:

- There really is no effect (association).
- There is a real effect but, by chance, the sample of people in the study did not show it.
- There is a real effect, which is seen in the study participants, but the study size (or number of events) was not large enough.

A p-value just above 0.05 (and ideally <0.10) could be interpreted in the same way as a 95% CI that just overlaps the no effect value, that is, there is a *suggestion* of an effect. P-values close to 0.05 (either just above or below) do not provide strong evidence either for or against an association [6].

There is a relationship between 95% CIs and statistical significance (using a p-value cut-off of 0.05). As the interval moves further away from the no effect value, in either direction, the p-value gets smaller (Figure 3.7).

3.4 Simple statistical analyses

The simplest types of analyses are used for comparing a single endpoint between two groups, and the exposure and outcome are each measured only once. Box 3.9 shows the most common methods, according to the type

---

Box 3.9 Simple statistical methods for comparing an outcome measure between two or more groups (e.g. exposed groups)

Type of outcome measure		Statistical test
'Counting people'	Outcome has ≥2 levels	Chi-squared (comparison of proportions)
		Mantel–Haenszel*
'Taking measurements on people'	Outcome is approximately Normal (Gaussian)	T-test (2 groups) Analysis of variance (≥3 groups)
	Outcome has a skewed distribution	Mann–Whitney test
Time-to-event		Logrank test

*Can allow for a few confounders using stratified analyses.

of outcome measure used. Some observational studies, particularly those that are quite small (e.g. <50 participants), are appropriate for simple tests. Further details about the statistical methods can be obtained from text books [7–9] or online sources [10]. These tests produce effect sizes, 95% CIs and p-values, and the focus of this book is on their interpretation and not how they are calculated.

When using 'counting people' endpoints to examine risk, a third factor (e.g. confounder) could be allowed for by considering each level of the factor as a stratum, and effects sizes (e.g. relative risk, risk difference, or odds ratio) are calculated in each stratum. The effect sizes are then pooled across all strata using the Mantel–Haenszel method (stratified analysis, which is analogous to taking a weighted average of the effect sizes across the strata) [7, 9]. A simple example is given in Figure 1.2b, where the relative risk for cirrhosis death is 1.0 for non-drinkers and 1.0 for drinkers, so the pooled (weighted average) relative risk will also be 1.0. A limitation is having many strata, some containing few individuals. This is also likely to occur when using two or more factors and each strata is a combination of every level of all the factors (e.g. if confounder A has 3 levels and confounder B has 5 levels, the effect size needs to be pooled across $3 \times 5 = 15$ strata).

3.5 Key Points

• Effect sizes compare two or more groups by combining the summary measures of outcome into a single number.
• There are various effect sizes: relative risk/risk ratio, absolute risk difference, and odds ratio for 'counting people' endpoints; mean difference for 'taking measurements on people' endpoints; and hazard ratio and risk difference for time-to-event endpoints.
• 95% CIs should be calculated for all main effect sizes.
• p-values (statistical significance) provide a measure of how likely the observed effect size could be due to chance in a study, assuming there really is no association.
• p-values ≥ 0.05 do not mean 'no effect' and those < 0.05 do not mean 'definitely an effect'.
• Although relative risk, odds ratio and hazard ratio are calculated differently, they can be interpreted in a similar way (all three uses risk)

References

1. Underwood B, Hackshaw A, Fox K. Smoking, alcohol and drug use among vocational dental practitioners in 2000 and 2005. Br Dent J 2007;203(12):701–5.
2. Doll R, Peto R, Boreham J, Sutherland I. Mortality in relation to smoking: 50 years' observations on male British doctors. BMJ 2004;328(7455):1519.
3. Espinosa PS, Kryscio RJ, Mendiondo MS, Schmitt FA, Wekstein DR, Markesbery WR, Smith CD. Alzheimer's disease and head circumference. J Alzheimers Dis 2006;9(1): 77–80.

4. Agnelli G, Verso M, Mandalà M, Gallus S, Cimminiello C, Apolone G, et al. A prospective study on survival in cancer patients with and without venous thromboembolism. Intern Emerg Med 2013. PMID: 23943559.
5. Royston P, Parmar MKB. The use of restricted mean survival time to analyze randomized clinical trials data when the proportional hazards assumption is in doubt. Stat Med 2011;30:2409–21.
6. Hackshaw A, Kirkwood A. Research and Methods: interpreting and reporting clinical trials with results of borderline statistical significance. BMJ 2011;343:doi:10.1136/bmj.d3340.
7. Kirkwood BR, Sterne JAC. Essential Medical Statistics. Blackwell Science. Second Edition (2003).
8. Petrie A, Sabin C. Medical Statistics at a Glance. Wiley-Blackwell. Third Edition (2009).
9. Bland JM. An Introduction to Medical Statistics. Oxford University Press. Third Edition (2000).
10. University of California, Los Angeles (UCLA) Statistics online help. Provides examples, with step-by-step explanations, and how to use statistical software for analyses. http://www.ats.ucla.edu/stat/stata/whatstat/. Accessed 16 May 2014.

CHAPTER 4

Regression analyses

The main limitation of most of the simple statistical methods in Section 3.4 is that they can only examine the relationship between one exposure and one outcome measure, each measured only once. In most observational studies, several factors are measured, or there could be several exposures of interest, and the aim is to examine these at the same time, including allowance for potential confounders. **Regression analyses** can do this easily, making them one of the most useful and common statistical methods for analysing observational studies. They come under the generic heading **generalised linear models** (the outcome measure, or some transformation of it, has a linear or straight line relationship with a set of factors) [1]. This chapter provides an overview of regression analyses.

Regression analyses may appear complex, but although the calculations would not be performed by hand, they produce the same effect sizes covered in Chapter 3, with 95% CIs and p-values, which are interpreted in the same way. There are other analytical methods, some more complex, and occasionally, it may be necessary to develop one for a particular study design and analysis, because of limitations of other methods, with 95% CIs and p-values, which are interpreted in the same way.

4.1 Linear regression

The following example highlights the general concepts underlying regression, using the simplest type, **linear regression** (or general linear model).

In a study in which blood pressure (outcome measure) and age (exposure) are determined on 30 men, aged 40–70, in England (see the scatter plot Figure 4.1), two questions are of interest:
1. Can the relationship be described and quantified in a simple way?
2. Can a man's blood pressure be predicted, given his age?

If there were no association at all between blood pressure and age, the observations would generally lie horizontally. However, Figure 4.1 shows a clear tendency for blood pressure to increase with increasing age, and it appears that a straight line could be drawn through the observations. There are mathematical

A Concise Guide to Observational Studies in Healthcare, First Edition. Allan Hackshaw.
© 2015 John Wiley & Sons, Ltd. Published 2015 by John Wiley & Sons, Ltd.

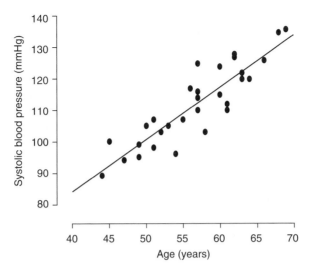

Figure 4.1 Scatter plot of 30 measurements of age and blood pressure.

techniques for finding the straight line that, on average, is closest to all the points: called the **linear regression line**.

The general form of a linear regression line is

$$Y(\text{outcome measure}) = a + b \times X(\text{exposure})$$

The regression analysis produces values for 'a' and 'b' (called **coefficients**):
- 'a' is the intercept and is the value of Y when X = 0. It often has no useful meaning on its own and is essentially used to help anchor the line.
- 'b' is the most important parameter, called the **regression coefficient** or **slope**. This is another form of **effect size** and is a measure of how much Y increases as X increases by a specified amount. In the example, Y (systolic blood pressure) increases by 17 mm/Hg as age increases by 10 years (e.g. from 50 to 60). This can be simplified to: as age increases by one unit (i.e. 1 year), blood pressure increases by 1.7 mm/Hg.
- If there were no association at all between age and blood pressure, a horizontal line would be observed, which has zero slope. This is the **no effect value** for a regression coefficient.
- Blood pressure increases with age, so the slope of the line is upwards; the regression coefficient has a positive value. If a regression line slopes downwards, the value of the outcome measure (Y) decreases as the exposure (X) increases, producing a slope with a negative value.

In the example, the form of the line is

$$\text{Systolic blood pressure} = 16.2 + 1.7 \times \text{age}$$

As with all summary measures, this line cannot perfectly represent all observations, that is, while some lie on or close to the line, others are far from it, such as the individual aged 54.

The equation can also be used to estimate the average level of blood pressure for any given age:
Age 50: average blood pressure = $16.2 + (1.7 \times 50) = 101$ mm/Hg
Age 60: average blood pressure = $16.2 + (1.7 \times 60) = 118$ mm/Hg
But this should only apply to men aged 40–70, for whom there were data in the analysis. Although a straight line fits the data in this age range well, the association could be quite different outside this range.

A linear regression model assumes that the observations are independent, and the following are each approximately Normally distributed: (i) the outcome measure (y-variable) at any value of the exposure (x-variable), and (ii) the residuals (observed value minus the value expected from the regression line). Sometimes, the outcome measure and exposure are each checked to determine whether they are Normally distributed (see page 30), and if either are clearly skewed, a transformation of the data is used before fitting the regression line.

What could the true effect be, given that the study was conducted on a sample of people?

The regression line comes from a *sample* of observations (30 men in the example), but the aim is to make inferences about the whole population of interest, that is, <u>all</u> men aged 40–70 in England. As with any other summary statistic or effect size, the regression coefficient (slope) will have an associated **standard error**, used to calculate a 95% CI:

$$95\%\text{CI for the slope} = \text{observed slope} \pm 1.96 \times \text{standard error}$$

The standard error for the slope in Figure 4.1 is 0.162, so the 95% CI is 1.4–2.0 (Box 4.1).

Box 4.1 Interpretation

The best estimate of the true slope is 1.7 mmHg, that is, this is how much blood pressure is expected to increase as age increases by 1 year.

It is not entirely certain that the true slope is exactly 1.7.

However, whatever the true value is, it is 95% certain that it should be between 1.4 and 2.0 mmHg*.

This range excludes a slope of zero, so there is confidence in the association being real.

---

*Technically, it is 95% certain that the range 1.4–2.0 will contain the true slope.

Could the observed result be a chance finding
in this particular study?
In the example, the p-value for the regression coefficient is <0.001. This means that if *it is assumed* that there really were no association (i.e. the true slope is zero, the no effect value), a slope as large as 1.7 or greater could be found by chance alone in <1 in 1000 similar studies of the same size. Therefore, the observed slope is unlikely to be due to chance, and so is likely to represent a real association between blood pressure and age. The p-value also allows for the possibility of the slope being −1.7 or lower (blood pressure decreases with increasing age), so it is a two-tailed p-value (as in Section 3.3), which is the most conservative and the one to interpret in most situations.

4.2 Identifying and dealing with outliers

Many observational studies are based on a large enough number of partici-pants so that a few overly large or small data values should not greatly influ-ence the results. Nevertheless, it is always worth checking the scatter plots for outliers. Figure 4.2a shows hypothetical data on blood pressure and age from 10 men, where there is no association (the slope is close to zero, 0.01). In Figure 4.2b, however, the presence of a single outlier creates a statistically sig-nificant negative association with slope −1.3. The line is trying to fit through all the data points, including the outlier, as best as it can, but as a result, it does not fit most of the observations. If data values like these are observed, they should be checked first to determine whether they are real or errors. If the value(s) is real, the regression analyses should be performed both with and without them, and the implications of both analyses should be discussed.

4.3 Different types of regressions

The type of outcome measure determines which effect size should be used, as well as the type of regression method (Box 4.2). These regressions all involve the same principle of trying to fit a straight line through something. This rep-resents the simplest association to find and describe. Linear regression involves fitting a line through a continuous (outcome) measurement, while logistic, Cox, and Poisson regressions do this through some measure of risk.

Risk can only take values between 0 (e.g. does not have a disorder) or 1 (does have the disorder), so the shape of risk in relation to an exposure varia-ble would look like Figure 4.3a; it can rarely be a straight line. This can be overcome by a transformation, using risk expressed as an **odds** (see page 51). A **logistic regression** analysis uses logarithm of the odds, $\log_e[\text{risk}/(1-\text{risk})]$, and the effect size it produces is an **odds ratio** (see page 51–52). With no upper or lower constraints, a straight line can be fitted, as with linear regression (Figure 4.3b). For time-to-event outcomes, the principle is similar to logistic regression, but $\log_e$ of the hazard rate is used, and this is analysed using a **Cox regression**, producing a hazard ratio. The interpretation of 95% CIs and p-values are as before.

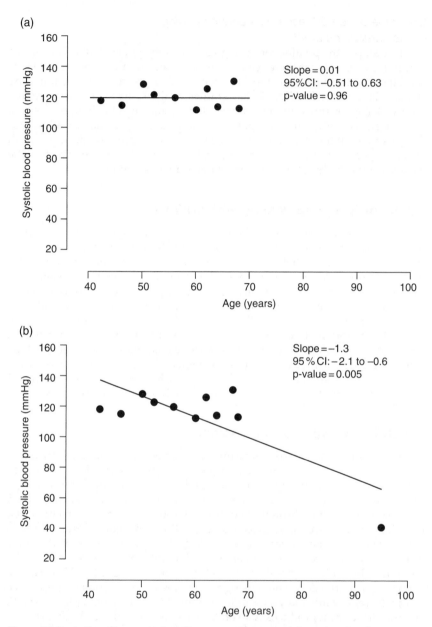

Figure 4.2 Illustration of how a single outlier can create an association, when the other observations do not show any association. The 10 observations in (a) are the same as in (b).

Box 4.2 Different types of regression analyses according to the type of outcome measure

Type of outcome measure (measured only once on each study participant)	Comments	Type of regression	Effect size produced
'Counting people'	• Binary (i.e. has only 2 levels, e.g. dead or alive)	Logistic regression	Odds ratio
	• Categories (≥3 levels) but with no natural ordering Ordered categories (i.e. has ≥3 levels) but with a natural ordering	Ordinal logistic regression	Odds ratio
	• Counting the number of individuals with or without an event, and they had different follow-up times*	Poisson regression	Relative rate
'Taking measurements on people'	• Continuous data (e.g. body weight, serum cholesterol)	Linear regression	Slope (regression coefficient), or mean difference
	• Counting the number of events per individual (e.g. number of days in hospital or number of asthma attacks)**	Poisson regression*	Relative rate
Time-to-event	• The time until a specified event(s) occurs (e.g. the time until death) or until date of last follow-up if it is not known whether the event has occurred	Cox regression	Hazard ratio

*If study participants start from a natural or defined starting point, then Cox regression can be used.
**Although based on events per person, the effect size produced is a relative rate, which can be interpreted in a similar way to a risk ratio, so it is more analogous to logistic or Cox regression than linear regression. But such outcomes could be analyzed using linear regression if there is a sufficiently wide distribution of events, though the effect size produced will be different.

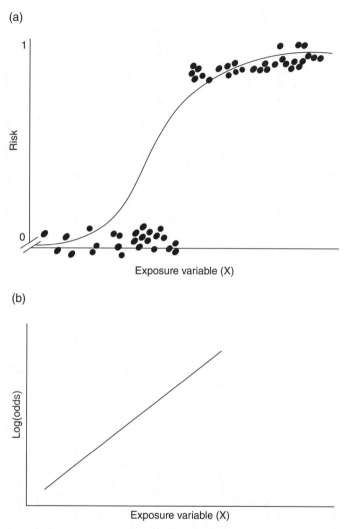

Figure 4.3 Illustration of how a straight line cannot be fitted through risk (a), but it can through the logarithm of the odds (b).

Each of the regressions in Box 4.2 produces an effect size. In the simplest case (one exposure and one outcome measure, each measured only once), they would be the same as those calculated by hand, for example:
* If observing the association between sex (exposure) and body weight (outcome), it is easy to calculate the mean weight among males and females separately and to take the difference (mean difference). This difference is identical to the regression coefficient **b** from the linear regression analysis of the data (weight = a + b × sex).

- If observing the association between sex (exposure) and heavy alcohol drinking (outcome), it is possible to summarise the data as a 2×2 table (Table 3.2A). The odds ratio is 3.9, and $\log_e(3.9)$ will be identical to the regression coefficient from a logistic regression analysis of the dataset (heavy drinker/not heavy drinker = a + b × sex).

Ordinal logistic regression

The simple logistic regression analyses presented earlier are based on a two-level outcome measure (e.g. dead or alive, developed disorder or did not, quit smoking or not). However, there are outcome measures with ≥3 levels, such as disease severity (none, mild, moderate, or severe). An easy approach is to collapse these into two levels, but information is then lost. Instead, an extension of logistic regression, **ordinal logistic regression** could be used. This produces odds ratios as before, but their interpretation is slightly different. Suppose the odds ratios in Table 4.1 came from an ordinal logistic regression where the outcome measure was severity of asthma among asthma patients: mild, moderate, or severe.

Suppose the exposure factor involves 'taking measurements on people' (continuous data), age:

As age increases by 1 year, the odds of being in a higher asthma severity group increases by 1.37 (37% increase) compared with all the lower severity groups. That is:

- *The odds ratio of having either moderate or severe asthma is 1.37, compared with having mild asthma.*
- *The odds ratio of having severe asthma is 1.37, compared with having mild or moderate asthma.*

If the exposure factor involves 'counting people' (categorical data), for example, sex:

The odds of being in a higher asthma severity group decreases by 0.75-fold compared with all the lower severity groups among females compared with males. That is:

- *The odds ratio of having either moderate or severe asthma is 0.75 (compared with having mild asthma) for females, compared with males.*
- *The odds ratio of having severe asthma is 0.75 (compared with having moderate or mild asthma) for females, compared with males.*

Table 4.1 Hypothetical results from an ordinal logistic regression, where the outcome measure has three levels (mild, moderate or severe asthma).

		Regression coefficient (odds ratio)*
Age (years)	1 year increase	1.37
Sex	Males	1.0
	Females	0.75

*Not on log scale.

A key assumption with this method is that the effect is the same across all categories of the outcome measure; otherwise, the same odds ratio cannot be used to compare higher categories with all lower ones (as in the descriptions given earlier). A **test of parallel lines** can be produced by the regression analysis to assess whether this assumption is correct. Also, if the outcome measure has many levels, a linear regression model might be more appropriate.

If the outcome measure has at least three levels, but there is no natural ordering to them, a **multinomial (polychotomous) logistic regression** could be used. One of the levels must be selected as the reference group, and an odds ratio is produced, which is the effect of each of the other levels, in comparison with the reference level. The interpretation of odds ratio is therefore not as simple as for logistic regression with a two-level outcome measure.

Poisson regression

Poisson regressions can be used for outcome measures that involve counts, including measuring risk of a disorder or death, for example:

- The occurrence of a disorder over a period of time
- The number of asthma attacks per patient during a year
- The number of days spent in hospital for each patient

The effect size is the **relative rate**, which has a similar interpretation to relative risk. Examples are shown in Box 4.3. Poisson regression can allow for different lengths of follow-up (exposure time) for participants.

A key assumption with Poisson regression is that the variance of the counts is similar to the mean value for each level of a factor being investigated. If the variance is much larger than the mean, this is called **overdispersion** and can occur when:

- There are outliers.
- There are missing data for the factors.
- Observations tend to cluster together.

Overdispersed data leads to standard errors, and hence p-values, that are too small (narrow 95% CIs). A **Pearson adjustment** could correct for the overdispersion; otherwise, more complex regression analyses should be used (e.g. **negative binomial**). But the same form of effect size is produced.

Multilevel modelling

Sometimes, the study has a hierarchical structure that may need to be allowed for, such as examining blood pressure between patients, and patients come from several hospitals; or the occurrence of a disorder based on individuals from different cities. Hospitals or cities would be called clusters. **Multilevel modelling** allows for these clusters by using random effects models, which can be done within linear, logistic or Poisson regressions. It estimates between-cluster variability and within-cluster variability. The effect sizes produced are the same as in previous sections, but the standard error of the effect sizes are often larger (than when ignoring the clustering) because it has allowed for two forms of variability [1].

Box 4.3 Examples of Poisson regression analyses

Outcome measure	Exposure factor	Regression coefficient (relative rate)	Interpretation
Number of days in hospital	Age (years)	1.04	As age increases by 1 year, the rate of hospital admissions increases by 1.04 (i.e. 4%)
	Gender (males vs. females)	0.66	The rate of hospital admissions is 34% lower among males than females
Occurrence of stroke	Blood pressure (mm Hg)	1.02	As blood pressure increases by 1 mmHg, the risk of stroke increases by 2%
	Smoking status (ever- vs. never-smoker)	1.45	The risk of stroke is 45% greater among ever-smokers than never-smokers

4.4 General comments on the different regression methods

Box 4.2 shows of the effect sizes produced by the different regression analyses. Researchers can get confused trying to remember what initially appears to be several distinct effect sizes and regression methods. However, the methods have common principles:

• The type of outcome measure determines which regression analysis should be used.

• The exposure factors (i.e. x-variables) can take any form out of continuous, binary, or categorical data; a time-to-event factor cannot be included unless every participant has had the event.

• The effect size for linear regression is usually a mean difference.

• If the exposure (or confounder) is a categorical factor (e.g. male/female, or never/former/current smoker), one level (e.g. male, or never smoker) must be chosen by the researcher and all comparisons are made with this group.

• The effect sizes for logistic, Cox, and Poisson regressions are always some measure of risk (or rate in Poisson) and can be interpreted in a similar way.

• The key difference between logistic and Cox regression is that logistic regression uses data that only indicates whether a study participant has had an event or not, while Cox regression incorporates the *time until* the event occurred.

4.5 Categorising exposure factors (variables)

When an exposure variable (or other factor) is based on 'taking measurements on people' (i.e. continuous data), it may sometimes be useful for interpretation to divide it into categories (see Figure 2.1). This can also make the data easier to show on a diagram. For example, categories that are familiar and easy to understand for age are 10-year bands: 20–29, 30–39, 40–49, and so on. Counting how many participants are in each category turns a continuous measurement into a categorical one. However, it is possible that some groups could contain too few participants to produce reliable effect sizes, or that researchers may deliberately define categories that tend to show the desired results. A more objective approach is to divide the data into **tertiles** (three groups), **quartiles** (four groups), or **quintiles** (five groups), which produces groups of almost equal size (see also Section 5.10 and Box 7.5). If the study is small, the division could be made above or below the median (i.e. 50% in each group).

If the data have been divided into tertiles, there will be two cut-off points that produce approximately a third of participants in each group. For quartiles there will be three cut-off points (~25% in each group), and for quintiles, four cut-offs (~20% in each group). Choosing the number of groups depends on the study size. Keeping the factor as a continuous measure uses all the data (information on variability is lost when dividing into categories), but this assumes that there is a linear relationship between the factor and outcome measure. It may be useful to analyse the factor in both ways to confirm that the conclusions are similar.

4.6 Interpreting p-values for factors that have ≥ 3 levels

When examining exposure factors that contain three or more levels in regression analyses, the interpretation of statistical significance requires care. Statistical packages automatically produce p-values for *each* level of the factor. Table 4.2 shows hypothetical results for three factors. The p-values for age and sex (0.03 and 0.02, respectively) should be used when assessing statistical significance. For smoking status (which has three levels), there are two p-values to consider (0.01 and <0.001), each compared with the selected reference category (never-smokers). These p-values test the effect of former and current smoking *separately*, but interest is really in smoking itself as a factor. The problem with interpreting several p-values for a single factor is that some could show statistical significance (<0.05), while others do not (≥0.05), making it difficult to reliably determine whether or not the factor is associated with the outcome measure.

A **change in deviance test** (under the general term **likelihood ratio tests**) will produces a single p-value for each factor. This p-value will be identical for age and sex (which are continuous or binary factors), as in Table 4.2. However, for factors that have ≥3 levels, such as smoking status, it will often be different from any of the individual p-values. The p-value in the example is 0.003, meaning that smoking status *per se* is associated with the risk of dying, and this is the p-value to interpret when making conclusions about the factor.

Table 4.2 The effect of three (exposure) factors on the outcome measure 'risk of dying'.

		Regression coefficient (odds ratio)	p-value	p-value from likelihood ratio test (logistic regression)
Age (years)	(1-year increase)	1.15	0.03	0.03
Sex	Males	1.0		⎫ 0.02
	Females	0.80	0.02	⎭
Smoking status	Never	1.0		⎫
	Former	1.50	0.01	⎬ 0.003
	Current	16.1	<0.001	⎭

Other likelihood ratio tests can be used for time-to-event or 'taking measurements on people' outcomes.

4.7 Examining several factors at the same time

The simplest regression model contains one exposure and one outcome measure, each measured only once, called **univariable** (sometimes **univariate**) **regression analysis**, but it is frequently necessary to examine several exposures at the same time. Also, many observational studies have exposed and unexposed groups with different characteristics, and allowance must be made for this (confounding). An example of adjusting for confounding was shown in Figure 1.2, when examining the effect of smoking on the risk of dying from cirrhosis, and alcohol drinking was the confounder. Separating (stratifying) the data according to drinking status is the simplest way to remove the effect of alcohol. If there were several confounders, the dataset would need to be divided into subgroups for every single combination of all factor levels, to ensure that each contains individuals with the same characteristics. But several subgroups are likely to be small, unless the study has a very large number of participants. Regressions efficiently allow for evaluating several factors simultaneously.

Multivariable (sometimes called multivariate) **regression** means that there are several factors (x-variables) in the regression model. They are just an extension of the univariable models presented earlier:

Linear regression:
Univariable: blood pressure = a + b × age
Multivariable: blood pressure = a + b × age + c × sex
Logistic or Cox regression:
Univariable: risk of developing heart disease = a + b × smoking status
Multivariable: risk of developing heart disease = a + b × smoking status + c × sex + d × gene Q

The mathematical details of how multi variable regressions work are not important here. What matters is that the effect sizes (odds ratio, hazard ratio, regression slopes, and mean differences) are interpreted in the same way as before, except that each estimate is *adjusted* for the effects of all other factors in the model. The factors could be a mixture of continuous or categorical variables. It is not possible to incorporate a time-to-event factor with censoring as an exposure factor. Examples of multivariable logistic, linear and Cox regressions are given in Chapters 5–7 and 9.

Occasionally, a regression analysis produces unusual results, such as extremely large or small effect sizes, or one end of a 95% confidence limit that is shown as infinity or 'not estimable'. This usually occurs when attempting to adjust for too many factors and the model cannot 'cope' because the sample size is too small, or when two or more factors are highly correlated. For logistic or Cox regression, the number of events is as important as study size; and as a guideline, there should be at least 10 events for each factor in a multivariable model in order to produce a sufficiently reliable analysis [2–4]. This is a guideline only, and not a strict rule [5].

4.8 Interactions between two exposures (effect modifiers)

When investigating the joint effect of two exposure factors on an outcome measure, multivariable regression analyses can be used to investigate (statistical) **interactions** between them. For example, a study could have the outcome measure 'proportion of smokers who quit smoking', and two factors of interest are age and sex. If there is no interaction, the relative risk for one factor will not depend on the other factor (Table 4.3).

In Example A in the table, even though the quit rates are higher for people aged ≥40, the relative risk for quitting smoking is 2.0 when comparing males with females, regardless of age group. There is no interaction between sex and age. In Example B, however, the relative risk is 1.0 (no effect) among people aged < 40, and 2.0 among those aged ≥40. There is evidence of an interaction: the effect of sex on quitting smoking depends on age. Age has modified the effect of sex on quitting and vice versa. This is referred to as **effect modification**, and sex (or age) is called an **effect modifier**. In Example C, the relative risk for sex is 2 and 5 for the younger and older age groups, so males are more likely to quit than females in both age groups, but the *size* of the effect is very different according to age (another interaction).

Table 4.3 Illustration of interaction for two exposure factors (age and sex) and an outcome measure (percentage of smokers who quit smoking).

	Age <40			Age ≥40		
	Males	Females	Relative risk*	Males	Females	Relative risk*
	Quit smoking (%)			Quit smoking (%)		
Example A	8	4	2	20	10	2
Example B	8	8	1	20	10	2
Example C	8	4	2	50	10	5

*% males/% females.

A statistical interaction is not the same as a biological interaction, which attempts to explain some underlying biological or chemical mechanism. Also, when evaluating a statistical interaction it should be made clear whether the conclusion is based on relative or absolute effects. In Table 4.3, the conclusions on interaction were made for relative risks, so there was no interaction in Example A. However, if absolute risk differences were examined, it would be +4 percentage points for age <40 and +10 percentage points for age ≥40; these are quite different, and it could be concluded that there was evidence of an interaction based on this type of effect size.

4.9 Measuring the outcome measure more than once during the study

The regression methods described earlier involve the outcome being measured only once, including endpoints that can occur only once, such as death or new occurrence of a disorder. **Longitudinal studies** are observational studies in which the outcome measure can be obtained from each participant on several occasions over time (e.g. measuring blood pressure, or the presence or absence of a characteristic such as asthma attack).

If the endpoint involves 'taking measurements on people' (continuous data) and there is only one measure at baseline and another later on during follow-up, the baseline value can simply be included in a multivariable linear regression as a separate factor. If it has been measured several times during follow-up, it is possible to use only the latest value (and again perform linear regression). However, if all the measurements are to be analysed, the statistical methods, which become more complicated, are those for **repeated measures analysis**. One example is **mixed modelling**. The format of the analysis looks very similar to multivariable linear regression, but it must be clearly indicated in the statistical software which set of data belongs to each participant. There are also various assumptions that could be made about the correlation structure of the outcome measure, that is, whether measures obtained far apart in time are less correlated than those close to each other. However, the effect size, 95% CI, and p-value produced are exactly the same as for linear regression, that is, a **regression coefficient or mean difference**, and interpreted in the same way.

If the outcome measure type is 'counting people' and there are only two levels (e.g. asthma attack or not, measured repeatedly over time), a **repeated measures logistic regression** can be used. An odds ratio is produced, as with simple logistic regression, but like mixed modelling, the data values that belong to each individual must be made clear in the statistical software.

4.10 Checking the regression model

A check of the goodness of fit (adequacy) of a regression model could be done, for example using residual plots (which essentially compare observed with predicted values from the model), or a Hosmer-Lemeshow test for logistic regression. Continuous measurements could be transformed (e.g. logarithms) to allow for very skewed factors, or grouped using justifiable categories if no suitable transformation can be found. If a linear model is not appropriate, more advanced methods, such as multi variable fractional polynomials could be used, which can fit various non-linear shapes to the association.

4.11 Missing data

Missing data is common, and is particularly troublesome in retrospective studies, where it is often impossible to obtain key data that have not already been collected. Missing data can significantly reduce the sample size for the statistical analysis, but there is also the potential for bias. Most regression analyses will ignore a participant if they have missing data for one of the exposure or confounding factors, even if the individual has data available for all other factors. If there are relatively few missing data (e.g. <5% of individuals are excluded from the analysis), this may not be a problem. If there are missing data for the outcome measure, these participants also cannot be included, although for studies that have repeated measures of the outcome, mixed modelling analysis and repeated measures logistic regression will only ignore the missing value at a time point (not all other time points). Cox regression will include data up to the time of last follow-up.

There are different categories of missing data, and each has implications for the analyses. But a key consideration is whether 'missingness' of a factor is directly related to that factor:

- **Missing completely at random**: As the term suggests, the missing data do not depend on any factor (including the exposure or outcome status of the individuals), in which case it should be acceptable to exclude these from the analyses, without affecting the conclusions.
- **Missing at random**: The missing data for a factor may depend on another factor, but not itself. For example, in a study to examine alcohol consumption, males may be more likely than females to not report their habits, but the 'missingness' should be random across the whole range of consumption. Sometimes, it is possible to ignore this form of missing data.
- **Not missing at random**: The missing data for a factor is related to the factor. For example, if considering alcohol consumption, if heavy drinkers were more likely to not report their habits, this would create a bias and so affect the results (e.g. underestimate the prevalence of heavy drinking). In this situation, missing data cannot simply be ignored, and statistical methods are required to deal with them.

There are various ways to address missing data, the best of which is to prevent it from occurring through good study design and by only collecting essential information. Another option is **sensitivity analyses**, which involves imputing (guessing) the missing data and examining how the results and conclusions change, though this requires various assumptions about the data and sometimes complex modelling (e.g. weighted estimated equations). One commonly used method is 'last observation carried forward', where a non-missing data value at, for example, 6 months is used as the 12-month value if the second value is missing. Although this is a simple approach, there are obvious problems, particularly if the time points are far apart, and so this method is not always recommended.

4.12 Key points

• Regression analyses are an efficient way of examining several factors (exposures) at the same time; but they produce the same effect sizes as in Chapter 3.
• The correct type of regression analysis (linear, logistic, Cox, and Poisson) depends on the type of outcome measure examined.
• It is useful to look for outliers, then examine their effect on the regression analyses.
• Missing data need to be explained, and consideration given to whether such data can be ignored or should be allowed for using statistical methods.

References

1. Kirkwood BR, Sterne JAC. Essential Medical Statistics. Blackwell Science. Second Edition (2003).
2. Peduzzi P, Concato J, Feinstein AR, Holford TR. Importance of events per independent variable in proportional hazards regression analysis. II. Accuracy and precision of regression estimates. J Clin Epidemiol 1995;48(12):1503–10.
3. Concato J, Peduzzi P, Holford TR, Feinstein AR. Importance of events per independent variable in proportional hazards analysis. I. Background, goals, and general strategy. J Clin Epidemiol 1995;48(12):1495–501.
4. Peduzzi P, Concato J, Kemper E, Holford TR, Feinstein AR. A simulation study of the number of events per variable in logistic regression analysis. J Clin Epidemiol 1996;49(12):1373–9.
5. Vittinghoff E, McCulloch CE. Relaxing the rule of ten events per variable in logistic and Cox regression. Am J Epidemiol 2007;165(6):710–8.

CHAPTER 5

Cross-sectional studies

5.1 Purpose

Cross-sectional studies are usually the simplest observational studies to conduct and analyse. They are often used to describe (summarise) the characteristics, habits, or opinions of a single group of participants. The results might then be used to explain findings from other studies, or help to design further studies. Cross-sectional studies are also used to examine the relationship between an exposure and an outcome measure, although this is often more reliably done using cohort or case–control studies. Sometimes, a sequence of cross-sectional studies over time (with almost the same design) could be used to examine trends in lifestyle habits, disease occurrence, or mortality. Further details on cross-sectional studies can be found elsewhere [1, 2].

5.2 Design

To ensure that the study objectives can be addressed satisfactorily, an appropriate **sampling frame** must be chosen (see Chapter 1, page 16). The choice of sampling frame will depend on how generalisable the results need to be, and on resources available to conduct the study (i.e. staff and money). The sampling frame also helps to define the eligibility criteria.

Box 5.1 shows four examples of sampling frames, based on studies summarised in Boxes 5.2–5.5 [3–6], discussed in this chapter. Key design features of these studies are shown in the boxes, which highlight similar aspects of cross-sectional studies in general.

The simplest sampling frame was the one based on children with terminal cancer [5] because it only required identifying participants from a single location (i.e. one hospital in Toronto), in which the research team worked. This is a common type of sampling frame, because it does not require significant resources (compared with studies that have regional or national sampling frames), and the conduct of the study can often be incorporated into the usual work of the research team. The VDPs sampling frame in Box 5.1 is also simple [3]. VDPs are one of several groups of people who are listed on a **regional** or **national register**, making it relatively easy to identify and contact them for participating in a study. Such registers can be a good way of obtaining regional

A Concise Guide to Observational Studies in Healthcare, First Edition. Allan Hackshaw.
© 2015 John Wiley & Sons, Ltd. Published 2015 by John Wiley & Sons, Ltd.

Box 5.1 Examples of sampling frames and how participants were selected from them

Study objective	Sampling frame (eligibility)	How were they selected
Describing the smoking, alcohol consumption, and drug habits of vocational dental practitioners (VDPs) [3]	VDPs registered in the UK, who started training in summer 2004	All were approached during January 2005
Examining the association between exposure to environmental tobacco smoke and chronic lung disease [4]	All adults from the registry of inhabitants in eight cities in Switzerland in December 1991	Random selection
Describing the quality of life (QoL) among children with terminal cancer [5]	Terminal cancer patients aged ≤18 seen between 2005 and 2009 at a single hospital in Canada	All were approached
Examining the association between dietary salt and blood pressure (BP) among adolescents [6]	A national survey on nutrition conducted in England, Scotland, and Wales in 1997 among children aged 4–18	Random selection

or national coverage. The other two studies in Box 5.1 use sampling frames that cover a wide geographical area, so would require considerable dedicated resources [4, 6].

Cross-sectional studies are often described as being conducted at 'one point in time', but the phrase is at best imprecise and at worst ambiguous. Two common meanings are:

1. All the data collected from a participant (e.g. lifestyle habits and characteristics) pertain to a single time point (actually a short time *period* such as a week or month), but the participants could have been identified over a short or long time period. The study on childhood cancer (Box 5.4) is an example of this. Each parent was interviewed only once about the QoL of their child, relating to the experiences around the time of the interview or recent treatment, but it took 5 years to accrue a sufficient number of subjects for a reliable analysis (2005–2009).

2. The participants are selected and data collected at a single point in time (again this actually could be a week or month), but some of the data

---

Box 5.2 Example of a cross-sectional study to describe the characteristics of a group of participants (outcome measure is based on 'counting people') [3]

Objective: To describe the smoking, alcohol consumption, and drug habits of vocational dental practitioners (VDPs), newly qualified dental graduates who must complete 1 year of training.

Study participants: 502 VDPs who started their vocational training in 2004 (out of 767 known to be in training).

Location: UK (all VDPs are on a national register, accessible through 77 VDP advisors).

Design: Anonymous questionnaire given to VDPs via their advisor in January 2005. To help ensure anonymity, age and ethnic origin were not recorded. The survey was distributed to VDPs by their advisor, during a study day, and took about 5 minutes to complete. The advisors then collected the questionnaires at the end of the session and posted them back to the study researchers.

Exposure: There was generally no concept of *exposure*, the main study aims were to examine the prevalence of certain habits, rather than associations.

Outcome measure: There were several outcome measures: (i) prevalence of current and ever smoking, (ii) alcohol consumption during the previous week and for an average week (from this, definitions of 'increased' and 'hazardous' were applied), and (iii) prevalence of current and ever users of recreational (including illegal) drugs. Results were presented separately by sex.

Results (among 502 responders): See Table 5.1 and Figure 5.1.

Authors' conclusion: Levels of binge drinking and cannabis use are relatively high in both men and women VDPs.

---

relate to lifestyle habits and characteristics that occurred in the near or distant past (e.g. several years before). An example is the study on chronic lung disease (Box 5.3), in which participants were selected at one time point (1991), but were asked about past exposures, such as parental smoking when they were children.

When the sampling frame and time period of recruitment have been determined, the process for selecting the participants, how this could be done, and who will administer the questionnaires or face-to-face interviews are decided. How participants are selected from the sampling frame depends on available resources and practicalities. In Box 5.1, two of the sampling frames were relatively small (VDPs, and children with cancer at one hospital), and the one for VDPs was also easy to access, so all were approached for participation in the study. However, in the other two examples (which have regional or national sampling frames of several thousand people), it was not possible to include them all, so a **random sample** was used instead. There are multiple methods for selecting random samples [7], but the ultimate purpose is to achieve a representative group from the sampling frame.

In the study of children with cancer, the clinicians and nurses identified and approached potential participants, and also collected the data. In the study of VDPs, all participants were under the guidance of a VDP advisor, to whom the

---

Box 5.3 Example of a cross-sectional study to describe the association between an exposure and outcome measure (outcome measure is based on 'counting people') [4]

Objective: To examine the relationship between passive smoking and chronic obstructive pulmonary disease (COPD).

Study participants: 4197 adults aged 18–60, who have never smoked.

Location: Eight cities in Switzerland, chosen to represent a range of urbanisation, altitude, air pollution, and weather conditions.

Design: Participants were selected randomly from the registry of inhabitants in each of the eight locations. Those recruited to the study were given physical examinations at a local research centre, where they also completed several questionnaires about their characteristics and lifestyle habits. The study was restricted people who had never used tobacco products or had smoked less than either 20 packs of cigarettes or 360 g of tobacco ever.

Exposure: 'Exposed' were never-smokers who had worked with smokers or had been exposed at home during the previous 12 months. 'Unexposed' are never-smokers without exposure at work or home.

Outcome measure: Chronic bronchitis symptoms (used to indicate COPD) defined as either coughing or bringing up phlegm on most days for at least 3 months each year for more than 2 years.

Results	Exposed never-smokers N = 1259	Unexposed never-smokers N = 2938
Cough/phlegm for ≥2yrs	98 (7.8%)	159 (5.4%)

Odds ratio (OR) for chronic bronchitis symptoms:

Crude (unadjusted)   1.47* (95% CI 1.14–1.91), p = 0.003

Adjusted (n = 3494)   1.65 (95% CI 1.28–2.16), p-value not reported

for age, sex, body mass index, geographical location, maternal and paternal asthma history, atopy, and asthma history of siblings.

Authors' conclusions: Passive smoking is associated with chronic respiratory symptoms.

*$1.47 = 98/(1259 - 98) \div 159/(2938 - 159)$

---

questionnaire packs were posted for distribution to the VDPs. In the studies of passive smoking and salt intake, which involved a geographical spread of participants too wide to be covered by the central research team themselves, staff were employed specifically for the study, to approach participants and/ or collect the data.

5.3 Measuring variables, exposures, and outcome measures

Central to any study design is the type and quality of data obtained. To ensure that the data are in an appropriate form to enable the study objectives to be addressed, the questionnaires should be carefully developed. If a questionnaire

---

Box 5.4 Example of a cross-sectional study to describe the characteristics of a group of individuals (outcome measure is based on 'taking measurements on people') [5]

Objective: To examine the QoL in children with cancer who have no reasonable chance of cure.

Study participants: Parents of 110 potentially eligible children aged 2–18. Thirty-seven could not be included because 13 died before parents could be approached, 3 were too unwell, 8 families were too emotionally overwhelmed, 1 was transferred to another hospital, and 12 families declined to participate. This left 73 parent/patient pairs available for the study.

Location: A single hospital in Toronto, Canada.

Design: Parent and children pairs were identified between June 2005 and October 2009 from the primary healthcare team of each patient. Children had leukaemia, solid tumours, or brain tumours. One parent (the main carer) was selected and interviewed in person while in the hospital or at home, during which time details about QoL were obtained. Other information (e.g. treatments received) was obtained from hospital records.

Exposure: Some analyses were descriptive; others examined the association between QoL and either (i) those who died ≤6 and >6 months after the parents were interviewed ('exposure' is timing of death) or (ii) patient characteristics ('exposure' was each of these characteristics).

Outcome measure: Three QoL instruments were used: (i) PedsQL 4.0 Generic Core Scales, which has 23 items and produces a total score and scores for physical, emotional, social, and school functioning; (ii) PedsQL 3.0 Acute Cancer Module, which has 27 items, covering 8 dimensions (pain and hurt, nausea, procedural anxiety, treatment anxiety, worry, cognitive problems, perceived physical appearance, and communication); and (iii) PedsQL Multidimensional Fatigue Scale, which has 18 items, covering general, sleep/rest, and cognitive fatigue. All scores are measured on a 0–100 scale.

Results: See Tables 5.2 and 5.3.

Authors' conclusions: Children had poorer physical health and more pain and fatigue when close to dying.

---

is being developed specifically for a study, it is good practice to first test the questions out on colleagues not involved in the study, or ideally potential participants. What might seem clear and obvious to the investigators might not be to others, especially the general public. The feedback often leads to questions being revised to improve clarity, making the questionnaire more 'user-friendly'.

Alternatively it may be possible to use standard questionnaires that already exist and have therefore been tested and validated. Box 5.6 lists several key general features of a good questionnaire.

The following sections illustrate some of the issues considered when developing questionnaires (or adopting standard ones), for the four example studies used in this chapter.

Box 5.5 Example of a cross-sectional study to describe the association between an exposure and outcome measure (outcome measure is based on 'taking measurements on people') [6]

Objective: To examine the relationship between dietary salt intake and blood pressure (BP) in children.

Study participants: 1658 children and adolescents aged 4–18, out of the total study population of 2672 children.

Location: UK. The participants were part of a national study (the National Diet and Nutrition Survey for young people).

Design: A national representative sample of 2627 participants was randomly selected from private households listed in the Postcode Address File (and only one child per household was included). Of these, 2127 completed an interview and had various measurements taken (including BP, body weight, and height) and a dietary record of all food and drink consumed over 7 days (including salt intake). 1658 children had both salt intake and BP available and were therefore included in the statistical analysis.

Exposure: Dietary salt intake was estimated by the researchers from the 7-day dietary record; it excluded salt added while cooking or at the table (the latter two were treated as separate factors in the analysis).

Outcome measure: The primary endpoint was systolic BP at rest, obtained after participants had not eaten or drunk anything for 30 minutes (the average of 2 BP values was used).

Results: See Tables 5.4 and 5.5.

Authors' conclusions: Increasing dietary salt among children is associated with increasing BP.

Box 5.6 Some key features of a good questionnaire

- Not too many questions.
- Unambiguous questions.
- Responses to a question consist of tick boxes covering several options instead of free text fields.
- Participants find it easy and relatively quick to complete.
- The questions have been used before, perhaps in other questionnaires, and so have already been tested and validated (i.e. they measure what they are supposed to measure).
- Define important terms, even if in common use (e.g. a unit of alcohol consumption or current smoker).

5.4 Collecting the data

Investigators can collect data in a variety of ways, depending on the study objectives and resources available (Box 1.9).

Face-to-face interviews and telephoning participants require members of the research team to undertake this often time-consuming activity (depending on the number of participants to be contacted), but a key advantage is that these approaches can significantly increase the response rate. Postal surveys can be a convenient way for participants to take part in a study, and to have greater coverage, but response rates can be relatively low (often <50%); using pre-stamped addressed envelopes usually improves this. Online surveys rely on participants having a computer at home and the software (database), which collects the data, being easy to use.

Random telephoning was, in the past, a common way of approaching potential participants, using listings of all home (domestic) telephone numbers in a regional or national area, or random digit dialling, which can be accessed after appropriate approvals have been obtained. However, many people (particularly young adults) now only have mobile telephones, so other methods have had to be developed to approach these as potential participants.

A balance must be achieved between trying to collect as much information as is required, and maximising the response rate. Response rate can be defined in a couple of ways: participants who complete some or all of the questions survey(s), or those who complete all of the questions. Participants faced with too many questions can be deterred from completing (or even starting) the questionnaire, or may rush through the questions and so answer some of them inaccurately (producing inconsistent responses to similar questions).

If the data collected directly from the participant are to be linked with other data (such as hospital records), the agreement and consent of the participant may be required, because the process is likely to involve the use of identifiers (such as date of birth and hospital number). Box 5.7 shows how different studies can collect data, using the examples in this chapter.

Box 5.7   How data were collected from the four examples in this chapter

Study	Methods of data collection
VDPs [3]	Anonymous self-completed questionnaire, distributed and collected by the VDP supervisors during classes
Passive smoking and COPD [4]	Self-completed questionnaire, and physical examinations conducted by research staff
QoL among young cancer patients [5]	Questionnaire completed by the parent of the participant, with additional data extracted from hospital records
Salt intake and BP [6]	Questionnaire completed by the participant or parent, and physical examinations conducted by research staff

---

Box 5.8   Simple approach to estimate sample size (N) for a single proportion (e.g. prevalence)

Example: Expected prevalence is $P = 65\%$

A 95% CI is required that has limits $\pm 10\%$ (i.e. it would be 55–75%):

$$95\% \; CI = 0.65 \pm 1.96 \times \text{standard error}$$

where standard error is $\sqrt{\dfrac{P \times (1-P)}{N}}$.

Rearranging this gives

$$N = P \times (1-P) \left(\frac{1.96}{\text{upper limit} - P} \right)^2$$

$$N = 0.65 \times 0.35 \left(\frac{1.96}{0.75 - 0.65} \right)^2 = 87 \text{ participants}$$

A table of sample sizes could be examined, covering a range of likely prevalence estimates, to see how study size changes with different estimates.

5.5 Sample size

Many cross-sectional studies do not have sample size calculations. This may sometimes be due to limited resources, for example, access to only a relatively small sampling frame (e.g. local hospital). In these situations, researchers may still want to pursue the study, because they would rather have some information than none, and are willing to accept that conclusions from a study that is not sufficiently large would not be strong.

If the aim of a study is to examine the prevalence of a disorder, or other type of event, a simple approach is to specify how narrow the 95% CI is required to be, and then work backwards to get sample size (see Box 5.8).

If the aim is to compare between exposed and unexposed groups, a similar approach to that for cohort studies could be used (Section 7.5).

5.6 Analysing data and interpreting results

The four examples in this chapter cover two of the types of outcome measured presented in Chapter 2:

1. 'Counting people' (binary or categorical data)
2. 'Taking measurements on people' (continuous data)

Examining time-to-event outcomes in cross-sectional studies is unusual (and often not possible), given the nature of the design, which does not involve any follow-up of participants over time. Also, cross-sectional studies cannot be used to estimate incidence rates, only prevalence.

It is useful to provide a table summarising the main characteristics of the study participants, and if there is an exposure of interest, these characteristics should be shown separately for exposed and unexposed individuals.

5.7 Outcome measures based on 'counting people' endpoints: Vocational dental practitioners (VDPs) and lifestyle habits (Box 5.2)

Measuring variables, exposures, and outcome measures

The main factors of interest in the study were the prevalence of smoking, alcohol consumption, and recreational (including illegal) drug habits of VDPs. These might intuitively seem easy factors to measure, but they each require careful definition so that the study participants answer the same question in a similar way. They are all self-reported measures, which rely on the participants to respond truthfully. Box 5.9 shows some examples of the questions used in the survey.

The definition of smoking is often given as one of three categories: current, former, and never-smoker, but these are not sufficiently specific to allow most participants to understand to which category they belong. The categories need to be defined more carefully on a questionnaire. A 'never-smoker' does not necessarily mean someone who has never smoked a single cigarette in their life; it might include those who have smoked a total of only <20 cigarettes their lifetime. This is a negligible amount, so such people could be included with those who really have never smoked at all. Formers smokers can be defined in many ways, for example, those who have successfully quit smoking for at least 5 years or perhaps a higher cut-off such as 10 years.

Alcohol intake is perhaps even more difficult to measure than smoking, partly because it is not something that many people consume every day. It was ascertained in several ways:

- Total number of units in the week previous to when the questionnaire was completed
- Total number of units during an 'average' week
- Total number of units during an 'average drinking session'

The first of these questions, being recent, should be the easiest to remember and should therefore produce more accurate responses, but might be influenced by the time of year. The researchers standardised this potential problem by distributing the questionnaires to all VDPs in mid-January, when it is expected that alcohol intake might be relatively low after the Christmas period, thereby giving conservative estimates of consumption. The other two measures aimed to ascertain the participant's typical or usual consumption, by asking for the 'average', but it might be difficult to recall this reliably, and there is likely to be variability in the interpretation of 'average'. A better study design would, in theory, have been to give the same questionnaire three or four times during the year to the same group of respondents (a longitudinal study). But without linking them to a particular individual, in order to maintain anonymity, which is essential here due to the sensitive nature of the

---

Box 5.9 Examples of questions used in the survey of VDPs

1. Which one of the following describes you **best**?
   a) I have never smoked tobacco. ❑
   b) I have tried smoking tobacco, but did not continue. ❑
   c) I smoke tobacco only while drinking. ❑
   d) I smoke tobacco only with cannabis. ❑
   f) I have been a regular* smoker as a VDP, but not now. ❑
   g) I currently smoke tobacco on a regular* basis. ❑

Regular = 10+ cigarettes per day.

2. How many units of alcohol did you consume last week?

1 pint of strong beer/lager	=3 units
1 pint of normal beer/lager	=2 units
1 bottle of alcopop	=2 units
1 glass of wine	=1 unit
1 measure of spirits	=1 unit

0–7	8–14	15–21	22–28	29–35	36–42	43–49	≥50
❑	❑	❑	❑	❑	❑	❑	❑

3. Which of the following (A–E) describes you **best** regarding your use of the substances below?
   A) I have never used this substance.
   B) I have used this substance once or twice.
   C) I have used this substance more than once or twice.
   D) I have been a regular user of this substance as a VDP, but I am not now.
   E) I am currently a regular user of this substance.

Please tick **one** appropriate box for each substance.

	A	B	C	D	E
i) Cannabis/marijuana* Hash, weed, dope, grass	❑	❑	❑	❑	❑
ii) Amphetamines** Speed or whizz	❑	❑	❑	❑	❑

*Regular = at least once a week.
**Regular = at least once a month.

---

questions. This would also require more resources. Using responses based on the number of alcohol units, one analysis involved grouping the participants into categories, one of which was 'binge drinking', defined as consuming at least half the recommended weekly limit in one session (which in the UK at the time was 21 units for men and 14 for women). Other researchers might not agree with the definition of a binge drinker, but what matters is that it has been clearly described in the published article.

A problem with all three measures of alcohol consumption is that they rely on the participant knowing how much alcohol constitutes a unit. Requesting this information in a more practical way, for example, by asking for the number of glasses of wine or beer, might yield more accurate responses, particularly because many people who drink alcohol underestimate their consumption. It is worth being aware how both the investigators and participants can create a bias. The investigators could change the cutoff for defining binge drinking, while a participant can misreport their alcohol consumption. Either situation can make the prevalence higher or lower.

Recreational drug use was the most sensitive factor requested (Box 5.9). It is unlikely that these are used as often as smoking or alcohol, so concepts such as a 'current user' and 'number of units' may not be readily comparable. In this study, VDPs were categorised as an 'ever user' if they had taken at least one of the specified drugs at any time while in training. A 'current user' was someone who had taken cannabis more than once or twice, or used it at least once per week, or used any other drug at least once per month. The definition of current user is clearly a mixture of habits, and it could be argued that a VDP who has only tried one drug on two occasions should not be grouped with someone who takes it every week. However, the nature of the habit and the potential for under-reporting suggest that, perhaps, a VDP who reports having taken a drug twice may have consumed it more often in reality. Again, the important principle is that the researchers fully define the groups.

When sensitive personal information is requested in questionnaires, the questions should be phrased carefully to maximise response and encourage truthful answers, be anonymous, and be reviewed and accepted by an **independent research ethics committee** (or **institutional review board**) (see Chapter 11, page 225).

Analysing data and interpreting results
What are the main results?
The main aim of this study was to examine the prevalence of various habits, rather than to make comparisons. Such descriptive studies, in require only summary measures for a single group of participants.

The data are summarised using a single percentage or proportion (see Chapter 2, page 28). **Bar charts** are a common and easy way to display such percentages. Figure 5.1 shows the results for current use of recreational (including illegal) drugs. Using percentages or proportions is better than using the absolute number, because they overcome differences in the denominators if comparing two or more groups (10 out of 20 is the same as 350 out of 700). The ordering of groups along the horizontal (x-)axis can be done in two ways. The first is to use a natural ordering, for example, severity of disease in four groups: none, mild, moderate, or severe (Figure 5.2). If there is no such ordering, as in the VDP study, the second method of ordering groups along the horizontal axis is by size of the percentage (largest one first). From Figure 5.1, we see that about 18% of males and 13% of females were ever users, but most of this is due to cannabis use.

Table 5.1 is an efficient way of presenting summary results for several endpoints (four in this example). It is unnecessarily repetitive to put the numerators in each cell or table, unless the denominators change. It is important to

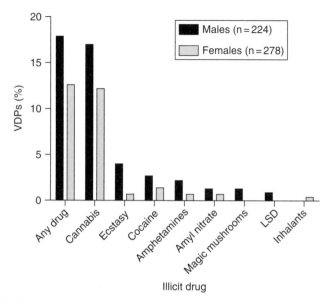

Figure 5.1 Bar chart showing the reported current use of recreational (including illegal) drugs among male and female VDPs separately. The bars are shown based on frequency of descending order. Current user is defined as someone who has taken cannabis more than once/twice, or uses it at least once per week, or uses any other drug at least once per month.

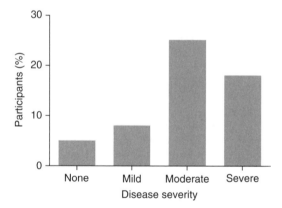

Figure 5.2 Hypothetical bar chart where there is a natural ordering to the categories (bars).

ensure that percentages add up to 100% (as in alcohol consumption). Missing data should be included as a row.

One question often asked is whether to put the percentage first or in brackets: '5.4% (12)' or '12 (5.4%)'. Because the percentages are the ones to interpret, it seems appropriate to make them prominent by placing them first.

The table can be used to describe the characteristics in each sex separately. Regular smoking appears similar between males and females, as does being a

Table 5.1 Selected key results on smoking, alcohol consumption, and drug habits among male and female VDPs [3].

	Males (n = 224)	Females (n = 278)
Regular smoker (≥10 cigarettes/day)	5.4% (12)	4.0% (11)
Alcohol consumption in an average week*		
Non-drinker	18.8% (42)	20.8% (58)
Sensible	55.8% (125)	66.6% (185)
Increased risk	24.1% (54)	11.5% (32)
Hazardous	1.3% (3)	1.1% (3)
Binge drinking**	44% (98)	39% (108)
Any recreational (including illegal) drug use		
Ever	38.8% (87)	27.0% (75)
Current	17.9% (40)	12.6% (35)

*Sensible drinking (recommended maximum): ≤21 units of alcohol for males and ≤14 for females, per week.
**Binge drinking: drinking half the recommended weekly maximum in one session (i.e. ≥10 units for males and ≥7 units for females).
Increased risk: 22–49 units for males and 15–35 for females.
Hazardous: ≥50 for males and ≥36 for females.

non-drinker, or hazardous drinker. More females were sensible drinkers, while more males were classified as having 'increased risk'.

What could the true effect be, given that the study was conducted on a sample of people?

The study was descriptive, so 95% CIs were not provided in the published paper. These could have been useful for some of the prevalence estimates, because the main purpose of the study was to describe the habits in all 767 UK VDPs, from whom a sample of 502 were analysed. CIs for percentages are easy to calculate (see Section 2.5). For example, the prevalence of binge drinking was 44% among males (98/224), with 95% CI 37–50%. Therefore, if all 767 VDPs had responded, the true prevalence would be expected to be somewhere between these two values.

Could the observed result be a chance finding in this particular study?

There is no concept of statistical significance when summarising the characteristics of a single group of people. If interest is in comparing one group with another, for example, binge drinking prevalence between males and females, then p-values could be calculated (See Box 3.2 and Section 3.3).

How good is the evidence?

Important features of the study design and conduct, and their potential impact on the results, are summarised in Box 5.10, along with those for the other three examples in this chapter, to allow a comparison.

Box 5.10 Examining the reliability of the study findings

Study	How good is the evidence: specific study features that should be considered when interpreting the results
VDPs [3]	• Fixed and known sampling frame (list of all UK VDPs), so it is possible to ascertain a good estimate of response rate • An attempt was made to include all VDPs, which is better than a random sample. Results likely to be generalisable • The questionnaires were sent in January, so participants could report recent habits, which might have been lower than usual, because of the post-Christmas period • The 35% non-responders could be more likely to have high consumption of smoking, alcohol, or recreational drugs; this could underestimate the prevalence estimates • Those with high consumption who did respond might have under-reported their habits • Anonymous questionnaire, so impossible to check whether general demographics differ between responders and non-responders (unlike the example of cancer patients below)
Passive smoking and COPD [4]	• Study participants were reported never-smokers, but this could include smokers who misreport their habits and so create a bias. However, the researchers addressed this by excluding 174 participants who had exhaled carbon monoxide levels ≥7 parts per million, which could indicate active smoking. The adjusted OR became 1.74 (1.65 originally) • Allowance was made for many potential confounders, so unlikely that important ones were missed • Additional confounders (to those in Box 5.3) were included, which reduced the sample size for the analysis to 2916, but the OR remained high (1.81) • There was consistency in the results for different respiratory symptoms (all but one had adjusted ORs showing increased risk among exposed never-smokers and are statistically significant) • A dose–response relationship was seen, where risk of having chronic bronchitis symptoms increased with increasing number of hours per day in which the participant reported having been exposed

	• Participants with respiratory symptoms may be more likely to report passive smoke exposure creating a bias (recall bias). However, the study was described as examining air pollution, with relatively few questions on passive smoke exposure
	• Participants came from various locations across Switzerland and various population types, so the results are likely to be generalisable within the country
Quality of life among young cancer patients [5]	• The response rate was 73 out of 110 (66%), which is reasonably acceptable. However, it could be that parents of the most ill children were more likely not to respond at this emotionally difficult time; this could bias the results
	• The sampling frame contained patient characteristics, so it was possible to compare these between responders and non-responders (no major differences were found)
	• The QoL symptoms were recorded in real time, so not affected by recall bias
	• The responses from parents were a proxy for the patient, and so may represent what the parents saw, rather than the actual experiences of the child
	• The analyses did not allow for any potential confounders, such as age, sex, or type of cancer, but the authors state that their study was intended to be descriptive only
	• The study was conducted in a single specialist hospital in Toronto. The findings might not be generalisable elsewhere, at either other hospital types or geographical locations
Salt intake and BP among adolescents [6]	• The study was based on national sampling of children and adolescents, so it is likely to be generalisable, certainly in the UK
	• It was a large study, in which many potential confounding factors were measured, and allowance could therefore be made for these
	• The estimated salt intake (exposure) was thought to be underestimated because it was not possible to reliably measure salt added during cooking or food at the dining table
	• BP (outcome measure) was assessed using a device not commonly used, and the device was known to produce higher values. However, this would apply to all study participants and should not materially influence the effect sizes

One key feature when assessing the quality of the evidence is whether the **response rate** is high enough. In this example, it is 65% (502/767), so the question is whether the responders are representative of all VDPs. The main problem in considering non-responders is that because they have not replied, researchers often do not know very much about them. Occasionally, it is possible to examine simple demographics of non-responders (e.g. sex and age), if they can be identified from the sampling frame.

It is difficult to determine what a 'good' or 'poor' response rate is, but clearly the higher, the better. Generally, 10% is probably poor and 90% excellent. What matters more than the percentage of responders is whether they have very different characteristics from non-responders, because it could influence the study findings if non-responders would have answered the questions very differently. If the characteristics of responders and non-responders were known to be similar, then a response rate of even 30% might be acceptable. The main implication of this would be to have wider 95% CIs, but the point estimates of prevalence should not be materially over- or underestimated.

In the study of VDPs, the 35% non-responders could have had very different smoking, alcohol and drug habits from the 65% responders. Those with high consumption might be more likely not to respond, and the effect of this **bias** is to underestimate the prevalence of these habits. Even though the survey was anonymous, VDPs who regularly took recreational drugs might still be wary of admitting to this, especially in a professional setting, and so not respond. Alternatively, those with high consumption might purposely underreport their habits, which would again affect the results. It is therefore certain that the true prevalence of binge drinking and cannabis was relatively high, because the estimates would be even higher than those observed if the assumptions above about the 35% non-responders are correct.

The findings were consistent with others studies of dental and law undergraduate students.

5.8 Outcome measures based on 'counting people' endpoints: COPD and passive smoking (Box 5.3)

Measuring variables, exposures, and outcome measures

This cross-sectional study (conducted in 1991) [4] was embedded within a larger longitudinal study (where the same subjects were reassessed in 2001–2003) (Box 5.3). Selected participants who agreed to take part in the study attended a clinic for various assessments (e.g. lung function), and completed a questionnaire asking about their characteristics, smoking habits, past exposures to tobacco smoke, and respiratory symptoms.

Because this study is an example of examining the effect of an **exposure** (passive smoking) on an **outcome measure** (a range of chronic respiratory symptoms),[#] each of these factors needs to be defined carefully and readily

---

[#] There were several outcome measures in the study, including wheeze, difficulty breathing, asthma, and chronic bronchitis; the last of these is used in this chapter.

captured on the questionnaires (Box 5.3). As with the example in Section 5.7, there are no perfect definitions of either the exposure or outcome measure. The exposed group relied on participants deciding whether they classified themselves as exposed, so may have included someone who had only been among smokers (i.e. exposed) once or twice during the year.

The investigators also wanted to adjust for the potential confounding effects of several factors, including age, sex, body mass index, geographical location, maternal and paternal asthma history, atopy, asthma history of siblings, and educational level, so the questionnaire had to be able to capture these data easily.

Analysing data and interpreting results
What are the main results?
The results for chronic bronchitis symptoms are shown in Box 5.3. The unadjusted (crude) OR is 1.47, so the chance of having these symptoms is 47% greater in the passive smoke-exposed group than the unexposed group.

An adjusted OR is also provided, allowing for the effects of various factors (Box 5.3). Comparing the unadjusted and adjusted estimates gives an indication of whether or not the factors were important confounders. In this example, the OR increased from 1.47 to 1.65. In many cases, the effect size to 1.0 (the no effect value), but occasionally, it becomes larger. Some of this increase will be due to chance, or random variation. What matters most is whether the effect of the adjustment significantly moves the OR closer to 1.0 (see also Figure 6.3). Both the unadjusted and adjusted estimates are always worth reporting.

The adjusted OR was based on 3494 out of 4197 participants. Although not discussed in the published paper, the difference of n = 703 should be due to missing data for some or all of the factors used in the adjusted analysis, and it would have been helpful if the authors had clarified this.

What could the true effect be, given that the study was conducted on a sample of people?
The 95% CI for the adjusted OR was 1.28–2.16. The true value is expected to be as low as a 28% excess risk, or as high as a doubling of the risk. The best estimate of the true effect, is 1.65.

Could the observed result be a chance finding in this particular study?
No p-value was provided for the adjusted OR of 1.65; however, it is possible to estimate it for the crude OR of 1.47 as p = 0.003 (using web-based calculators or freely available software [8]). Because the adjusted estimate is larger than 1.47 and the lower end of the 95% CI further away from 1.0 (see Figure 3.7), it is likely that the p-value for 1.65 is <0.003[#]. Both are statistically significant. If it is assumed that there really was no association between passive smoke exposure and chronic bronchitis symptoms, that is, the true OR is 1.0, then we expect to see an effect as large as 1.47 or greater, or the same size of effect in the opposite direction (i.e. 1/1.47 = 0.68 or lower), in only 3 in 1000 similar

---

[#]It is <0.001 using Box 6.8

studies of the same size, just due to chance. Therefore, the observed result is unlikely to be due to chance; it is likely to be a real effect.

How good is the evidence?
Box 5.10 provides some general comments on features of this study that should be considered when interpreting the results. The study was based on a random selection of residents in each Swiss location, of whom 59% were recruited to the study (response rate).

As with any cross-sectional study, a range of factors could influence the association between the exposure and outcome measure. In the example, potential confounders included physical characteristics (e.g. age, sex), and exposure during childhood. There may also be other confounders that cannot be allowed for in the statistical analysis, because they had not been measured.

The findings were consistent with other studies on chronic bronchitis and passive smoke exposure, which provides further supporting evidence for a real association.

5.9 Outcome measures based on 'taking measurements on people' endpoints: Quality of life in young cancer patients (Box 5.4)

Measuring variables, exposures, and outcome measures
The outcome for the study shown in Box 5.4 might initially be thought to be 'cancer'. However, the purpose of the study is actually to determine the effect of having cancer on QoL measurements. Therefore, having cancer is the exposure, and the outcome measure is QoL.

Various characteristics of the parents and cancer patient were collected for each participant, including the child's age and gender, educational level of the parent, and details about the cancer (e.g. type of cancer, and number of years since diagnosis). This study was also used to examine the relationship between an exposure (parent and child characteristics) and outcome (QoL).

For certain study outcomes, it is best to use a questionnaire that has already been developed and accepted for use, especially when assessing and measuring factors such as QoL which can be complex. The investigators of the cancer patients study used three established questionnaires (also called instruments); Box 5.4.

Other disorders have specific QoL instruments, for example, the Barthel Index for stroke patients [9] or Dementia Quality of Life Instrument (DQoL) for people with dementia [10]. For general public use, the Short Form 12 or 36 [11] are often used. Using an existing validated questionnaire will save time and resources, although there will be circumstances where the investigators must develop their own, and sufficient time should be allowed for this.

Analysing data and interpreting results
What are the main results?
The outcome measure (QoL) was analysed using either a t-test or **linear regression** (see pages 63 and 66).

Table 5.2 Selected QoL results according to timing of death.

	Mean QoL score*			
	Died ≤6 months after interview (n=30)	Died >6 months after interview (n=43)	Mean difference*, B−A (95% CI)	p-value
	A	B		
Generic core scales				
Total	45.8	53.1	7.3 (−2.6, 17.2)	0.15
Physical summary	32.8	48.6	15.9 (1.8, 30.0)	0.028
Psychosocial summary	54.2	56.0	1.8 (−6.9, 10.6)	0.68
Acute cancer module				
Pain and hurt	45.0	60.5	15.5 (0.9, 30.0)	0.037
Procedural anxiety	43.3	58.1	14.8 (−0.8, 30.4)	0.062
Worry	69.8	66.5	−3.4 (−17.1, 10.3)	0.63
Fatigue scale				
General	38.3	54.1	15.8 (2.4, 29.1)	0.021
Sleep/rest	46.4	62.4	16.0 (3.5, 28.5)	0.013

*High score is associated with better QoL; so a positive mean difference indicates that children who died >6 months after interview had better scores than those who died ≤6 months after interview.
The mean difference, 95% CI, and p-values come from a t-test.

In this study, the outcome measure involved obtaining QoL scores from the participants. One analysis aimed to compare the scores between patients who died within or after 6 months following the interview. Table 5.2 shows the mean (average) scores in each group. This type of outcome measure ('taking measurements') should always be interpreted using the scale of the measurement. Here, each score ranges from 0 (worst health) to 100 (best health). The mean scores (about 40–60) show moderate health, but these are averages, so there will be some individual patients who had lower or higher scores than the mean values shown. Patients who died within 6 months of the interview seemed to suffer most on physical health (mean = 32.8) and general fatigue (mean = 38.3) scores, as these were the lowest mean scores.

The effect size for this type of endpoint is the difference between the two mean scores. The differences ranged from being small ('psychosocial', mean difference = 1.8) to moderate ('sleep/rest', mean difference = 16.0). It is worth attempting to describe observed effect sizes as small, moderate, or large, to help interpretation, even though this crude categorisation will often be subjective.

Table 5.3 shows the results for the association between one patient characteristic (age) and one measure of QoL (physical), using linear regression analyses. There would be a separate regression analysis for each of the eight QoL

Table 5.3 Linear regression analyses between age (exposure) and 'physical' QoL outcome measure.

Age (years)	No. of patients	Slope* (SE)	p-value
2–4	8	9.86 (12.60)	0.44
5–7	22	15.46 (9.20)	0.10
8–12	21	3.93 (9.31)	0.67
13–18	22	Reference	

SE, standard error.
*That is, regression coefficient.

measures in Table 5.2. The effects sizes (slopes) appear completely different from those in Table 5.2, but in fact they have the same interpretation.

When the exposure factor has two groups, the data can be analysed using a two-sample t-test. When the factor has three or more groups, three separate t-tests could be performed for each pair, but this is inefficient, and each p-value does not take into account that two other comparisons have been made. A regression analysis will use all data at the same time. The effect size is called the **slope** (see Section 4.1), but in Table 5.3, one age group (13–18) has been labelled the 'reference' group. The slope is simply the mean difference between each age group and the reference. For example, the slope among ages 2–4 is 9.86. This is the mean score for patients aged 2–4 minus the mean score for those aged 13–18 (similar to the mean differences in Table 5.3). Generally, the slopes (mean differences) are positive, indicating that, on average, younger patients had better QoL symptoms than the oldest age group, ranging from small (mean = 3.93) to moderate (mean = 15.46) differences.

The lowest category is often chosen as the reference group, but the highest group is used in the example, probably because it contains more patients than the 2–4-year age group.

What could the true effect be, given that the study was conducted on a sample of people?

From Table 5.2, the 95% CIs were generally wide, which is not surprising given the study size of only 73 participants. Several fields ('total', 'psychosocial', and 'worry') contain the no effect value (mean difference of zero), indicating the possibility that there could be no real difference in the mean scores between the two groups, or small effects.

There were eight factors in the table, each analysed separately. To help address having multiple comparisons,[#] researchers could consider providing 99% CIs [12].

[#] The more comparisons examined, the more likely that some will be found to be statistically significant but are really due to chance.

Could the observed result be a chance finding in this particular study?
In Table 5.2, no result was highly statistically significant (p < 0.001), and the strongest evidence was seen for 'general fatigue' and 'sleep/rest', because they had the smallest p-values of those shown (0.021 and 0.013).

Little evidence of an effect is seen for the generic core scale 'total' and 'psychosocial', because the p-values clearly exceed p = 0.05, and the effect sizes are small and close to the no effect value of zero.

One result ('procedural anxiety') had a p-value of 0.062, which just exceeds the conventional level for statistical significance (p = 0.05), but the effect size had a similar magnitude to 'fatigue'. It would not be correct to conclude that there was no association with 'procedural anxiety'. It is likely that there was more variability in this outcome measure (i.e. greater standard deviation), and that this contributed to the slightly larger p-value.

In Table 5.3, a p-value is given for each comparison with age 13–18. These values will be higher than those produced by separate t-tests, because they all come from a single regression, and so have essentially allowed for multiple comparisons (corresponding to the three age groups). However, these p-values can only be used to examine the effect within a specific age category, and it would have been more useful to show the <u>overall</u> p-value for age, which addresses the question of whether there is an association *per se* between age and QoL among these patients (see Section 'Interpreting p-values for factors that have ≥3 levels', page 76). For 'physical', the effect sizes are 9.86, 15.46, and 3.93 as age increases, which shows no obvious monotonic increase or decrease. The conclusion is that, although these scores tend to be better among younger patients, there is no clear evidence for a trend.

How good is the evidence?

Box 5.10 shows some general aspects of the study relevant for interpreting the results. This was the first large study to comprehensively examine QoL among terminally ill children with cancer. Given the sensitive nature of the subject, it was important to approach parents and administer the questionnaires with great care.

The 66% response rate was acceptable, and because the sampling frame contained patient characteristics, it was possible to compare age, sex, and type of cancer between responders and non-responders. No material differences were found.

All of the statistical analyses were univariable, so they did not allow for other potential confounding factors at the same time. Therefore, some of the associations found might not have been real. The researchers acknowledged this in their discussion and noted that the study was intended to be largely descriptive. The value of the 95% CIs might be less important in studies such as this one, but researchers are now accustomed to providing them, and journal editors frequently request them.

The authors examined the few other published studies on this subject, and it was possible to show consistency in comparable QoL scores, particularly in patients surviving for more than 6 months.

5.10 Outcome measures based on 'taking measurements on people' endpoints: Salt intake and blood pressure among adolescents (Box 5.5)

Measuring variables, exposures, and outcome measures

In the study shown in Box 5.5, dietary salt intake (the exposure) was estimated using a 7-day dietary record of all food and drink consumed by the participants. This was completed by the parent if the child was not old enough. Salt is contained in many foods, so it was not possible for the participants themselves to estimate their intake. The investigators made these estimations using the detailed information provided by the participants, which was converted to grams per day and averaged over the week. It is possible that the physical act of measuring each food item might have increased parental awareness of what they were giving their children, and that they therefore changed their habits during the study.

The outcome measure (BP) was assessed by a member of the research team who visited the home. Other characteristics obtained included gender and body weight, which were easy to measure.

Analysing data and interpreting results

What are the main results?

A simple diagram for the presentation of the type of data collected in this study would have been a scatter plot of BP (y-axis) against salt intake (x-axis), to show if there was a trend going either up or down, but such a plot was not provided in the published article. When there are several hundred or more observations, one issue over scatter plots is overlapping points, although there are graphic packages that can separate these points out. Instead of a diagram, the authors of the salt intake paper provided many summary results in a single table (including sex, age, salt and sodium intakes, body mass index, and BP), using the mean values and standard error of the means.

Salt intake (the exposure, Table 5.4) was categorised into three groups (for each age group) using tertiles (see page 76). For example, there were 553 children aged 4–8, so there will be two salt intake values that divide them into three groups with approximately n = 184 in each (553/3): there were n = 184 with intake <4.6 g/day, n = 185 with intake between 4.6 and 5.5 g/day inclusive, and n = 184 with intake >5.5 g/day.

Figure 5.3 was derived using the summary results (mean BP and standard errors) contained in one of the tables in the article.[#] Such diagrams can help to communicate easily the main findings of a study. The figure shows instantly that within each age group, BP increases with increasing tertile of salt intake. It is also clear that systolic BP increases with increasing age. Table 5.4 shows that salt intake also increases with increasing age, so age is a confounding

---

[#]For example, among children aged 4–8, the mean systolic BP in the first tertile was 101 mmHg, with standard error 0.6; so the lower and upper 95% CI limits (shown in Figure 5.3) are $101 \pm 1.96 \times 0.6$, which is 100–102.

Table 5.4 Mean salt and sodium intake and systolic BP in each tertile of salt intake (in each age group).

	Aged 4–8 years			Aged 9–13 years			Aged 14–18 years		
Tertile of	1	2	3	1	2	3	1	2	3
salt (g/day)	<4.6	4.6–5.5	>5.5	<5.5	5.5–6.7	>6.7	<5.7	5.7–7.5	>7.5
No. of children	184	185	184	203	203	203	165	166	165
% boys	41	58	64	34	50	67	19	46	77
Mean salt intake (g/day)	3.8	5.0	6.6	4.5	6.0	7.9	4.5	6.5	9.3
Mean systolic BP (mmHg)	101	103	103	107	107	109	112	116	119

Observations:
- The number of children in each salt intake group is similar (in each age group), because tertiles were used.
- The percentage of boys is greater in tertiles 2 and 3 than tertile 1.
- Salt intake increased across tertiles (as must happen, because of the way tertiles were defined).
- BP appears to increase with salt intake and also with age.

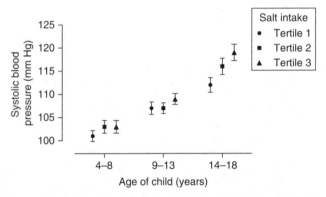

Figure 5.3 Diagram showing how the mean systolic BP (and 95% CI) changes with tertile of dietary salt intake, according to age group (the tertile categories are shown in the header of Table 5.5). An alternative figure is to display all the individual BP values, with the mean and standard deviations (or median and interquartile range) indicated; this would show the actual data, while the figure shows a summary of the data.

factor, when examining the association between BP and salt, and that there were more boys in the higher salt intake categories.

The results of a linear regression analysis are provided in Table 5.5. In the published results, all factors included simultaneously in the analysis were shown in a table, but for simplicity, only salt intake, age, and sex are given here. The effect size is the **regression coefficient** (or slope; see Chapter 4, page 67), and the no effect value is zero. BP increased by:
- 0.40 mmHg as salt intake increased by 1 g/day.
- 0.86 mmHg as age increased by 1 year.

Table 5.5 Linear regression analyses between systolic BP (outcome) and three exposure.

	Coefficient (SE)*	95% CI**	p-value
Salt intake (g/day)	0.40 (0.17)	0.07–0.73	0.018
Age (years)	0.86 (0.07)	0.72–1.00	<0.001
Sex	2.06 (0.49)	1.10–3.02	<0.001

*Adjusted for all the other factors in the table plus potassium intake and body mass index.
**The 95% CIs were not given in the article, but they are easily calculated by hand using the reported coefficient and standard error (SE): 95% CI = coefficient ± 1.96 × SE.

- 2.06 mmHg as sex 'increased by 1 unit', but sex has only two categories (probably coded as 1 = male and 0 = female), so a difference of 1 unit is actually just the difference in mean values between males and females; that is, BP in males is, on average, 2.06 mmHg higher than in females.

Each of the above effect sizes were adjusted for all other factors included in the model, including potassium intake and body mass index. The adjusted effect size indicates that salt intake has an *independent* association with BP (i.e. it is not influenced by the four other factors in Table 5.5).

The clinical importance of the association between salt intake and BP could be considered in relation to a recommended daily maximum intake for UK children: 3 g for those aged 4–8, 5 g for 7–10, and 6 g for ≥11 [13]. In the study, the mean salt intake ranged from 3.8 to 9.3 g/day across the age groups (Table 5.4), so an increase of 1 g is significant. However, this is associated with an average increase in BP of only 0.4 mmHg, which is a small effect considering that the mean values range from 101 to 119 mmHg (Table 5.4). The public health impact is that, perhaps, a high salt intake at a young age can persist into adulthood, and therefore have longer term implications on hypertension and cardiovascular disease. In comparison, the effect on BP was greater for age and greatest for sex; both regression coefficients (0.86 and 2.06) were larger than that for salt intake (0.4).

What could the true effect be, given that the study was conducted on a sample of people?

In Table 5.5, the 95% CI indicates that the true increase in BP associated with an increase of salt intake of 1 g/day is expected to be between 0.07 and 0.73. The lower limit is a very small effect, although it exceeds the no effect value of 0, but even the upper limit does not represent a major change in BP.

Could the observed result be a chance finding in this particular study?

The small effect size (0.40) from a large study, produced a p-value of 0.018. This is below 0.05, but not very small (see Figures 3.5 and 3.7). Therefore, while it is possible to conclude that there is likely to be a real association, the evidence is modest. The p-values for age and sex provide stronger evidence for an association because they are smaller (< 0.001).

How good is the evidence?
Box 5.10 shows some general comments of this study. The study was relatively large and has therefore shown some clear associations, although considered as small effects. However, salt intake was only measured over a very short time period (7 days), and not over a year which would show how intake changes over time within an individual.

The association between salt intake and BP among adults is well established, so it is plausible to have a similar association in children. The result (an increase of 0.4 mmHg for an extra 1 g/day of salt) is consistent with a meta-analysis of 10 clinical trials of children and adolescents [14], in which BP decreased by 1.2 mmHg for an average decrease of salt intake of 3 g/day (which is 1.2/3 = 0.4 mmHg for 1g, as observed in the cross-sectional study). Further supporting evidence comes from experimental studies of primates, which showed clearly that BP increased as salt intake increased, (and this could be considered cause and effect, due to the experimental nature of this particular study).

5.11 Key points

• There can be several definitions of cross-sectional, and such studies are a relatively quick and easy way to examine the characteristics of a single group of people, or associations between factors and outcomes.
• Specification of the sampling frame is essential and will help determine whether the results and conclusions are generalisable to the target population of interest.
• Participants should not be selected from the sampling frame in a way that could create bias (so that the results are significantly under- or overestimated).
• It is best to use established (validated) questionnaires; otherwise, resources should be available to properly develop new ones.
• Questions in the questionnaires must be clear and unambiguous so that participants read and interpret them in a similar way (acknowledging that many factors do not have a single, established definition).
• Data can be collected in several ways; the choice may depend on the type of information to be collected.
• Response rates should be sufficiently high, and consideration given to whether non-responders would have provided very different results to the responders (creating bias).
• The interpretation of effect sizes such as relative risk, OR, and mean difference (and 95% CIs and p-values) is the same as in other chapters.

References

1. dos Santos Silva I. Cross-sectional surveys. In: Cancer Epidemiology: Principles and Methods. IARC Press (1999). http://www.iarc.fr/en/publications/pdfs-online/epi/cancerepi/. Accessed 15 May 2014.
2. Silman AJ, Macfarlane GJ. Epidemiological Studies: A Practical Guide. Cambridge University Press. Second Edition (2002).

3. Underwood B, Hackshaw A, Fox K. Smoking, alcohol and drug use among vocational dental practitioners in 2000 and 2005. Br Dent J 2007;203(12):701–5.
4. Leuenberger P, Schwartz J, Ackermann-Liebrich U, Blaser K, Bolognini G, Bongard JP, et al. Passive smoking exposure in adults and chronic respiratory symptoms (SAPALDIA Study). Swiss Study on Air Pollution and Lung Diseases in Adults, SAPALDIA Team. Am J Respir Crit Care Med 1994;150(5 Pt 1):1222–8.
5. Tomlinson D, Hinds PS, Bartels U, Hendershot E, Sung L. Parent reports of quality of life for pediatric patients with cancer with no realistic chance of cure. J Clin Oncol. 2011; 29(6):639–45.
6. He FJ, Marrero NM, Macgregor GA. Salt and blood pressure in children and adolescents. J Hum Hypertens 2008;22(1):4–11.
7. Moser C, Kalton G. Survey Methods in Social Investigation. Dartmouth Publishing Co. Second Edition (1985).
8. Epi Info, Version 7. US Centers for Disease Control and Prevention. http://wwwn.cdc.gov/epiinfo/7/. Accessed 15 May 2014.
9. Shah S, Vanclay F, Cooper B. Improving the sensitivity of the Barthel Index for stroke rehabilitation. J Clin Epidemiol 1989;42(8):703–9.
10. Brod M, Stewart AL, Sands L, Walton P. Conceptualization and measurement of quality of life in dementia: the dementia quality of life instrument (DQoL). Gerontologist 1999;39:25–35.
11. Short Forms 12 or 36. http://www.qualitymetric.com/. Accessed 15 May 2014.
12. Altman DG, Machin D, Bryant TN, Gardner MJ. Statistics with Confidence. BMJ Books. Second Edition (2000).
13. Salt and Health. Scientific Advisory Committee on Nutrition. Her Majesty's Stationery Office, 2003. http://www.nhs.uk/livewell/goodfood/pages/salt.aspx. Accessed 15 May 2014.
14. He FJ, MacGregor GA. Importance of salt in determining blood pressure in children: meta-analysis of controlled trials. Hypertension 2006;48(5):861–9.

CHAPTER 6

Case–control studies

6.1 Purpose

Case–control studies are generally considered to be the next most reliable study design after cohort studies when evaluating risk factors and causality (Chapter 1, page 13). Further details on case–control studies can be found elsewhere [1–4].

6.2 Design

Case–control studies specifically involve selecting participants based on a disease or event status (Figure 6.1). They are therefore usually designed with a particular disorder in mind, with participants classified as with or without the disorder (i.e. cases or controls), or to include mortality (dead or alive). However, event status could be used for any defined feature, for example, quit smoking (cases) or not (controls), or leaves hospital within 30 days (cases) or not (controls). Case–control studies are particularly useful when the outcome is relatively rare, making a prospective cohort study unfeasible because there would need to be an impractically large number of participants followed up for a long time before a sufficient number develop the disorder of interest (Box 1.7).

As with all observational studies, a sampling frame needs to be defined. However, unlike cross-sectional and cohort studies, which usually have a single sampling frame, case–control studies can have two different sources, one for cases and another for controls. Box 6.1 shows three examples, used in this chapter (Boxes 6.2–6.4) [5–7]. The boxes show key features of how the studies were conducted, including exposures and outcomes, and these highlight similar aspects to consider when examining case–control studies in general.

Selecting the cases

Identifying cases can be relatively straightforward, with an obvious sampling frame to work from. They could be found from hospital/clinical records and databases, a network of health researchers, disease registries, notification

---

A Concise Guide to Observational Studies in Healthcare, First Edition. Allan Hackshaw.
© 2015 John Wiley & Sons, Ltd. Published 2015 by John Wiley & Sons, Ltd.

Box 6.1 Examples of sampling frames and how participants were selected from them

Study objective	Sampling frame (eligibility) and how they were selected	
	Cases	Controls
To examine the association between sleeping environment of infants and the risk of sudden infant death syndrome (SIDS) [5]	• Three National Health Service regions in the UK, in which there was a network of professionals and lay organisations that reported all sudden unexpected deaths within 24 hours. • The researchers also found cases through the national notification registry. • All mothers who had an affected infant were approached if the death occurred from either February 1993 (two regions) or September 1993 (one region) until January 1995.	• The health visitor of each case of SIDS selected four babies on his/her assigned list: two who were the next older and two the next younger. • If all four were not available, the baby with the next closest age was chosen; and if this failed, the health visitor selected from his/her nearest colleague's list. • Controls were therefore matched for age and geographical location.
To examine the relationship between head circumference and Alzheimer's disease [6]	• Patients diagnosed with Alzheimer's disease at a single specialist centre in Kentucky, US. Patients after March 1992 were selected, because this was when head circumference was routinely measured. • Patients had to be ≥60 years old (to use the control group from the same centre).	• Healthy volunteers participating in a research project at the same specialist centre, who were ≥60 years old at baseline. • There was no matching.
To examine whether survival is different between cancer patients with and without venous thromboembolism (VTE) [7]	• Patients with advanced solid cancer attending 1 of 51 cancer centres in Italy up to December 2009. To be eligible, they had to have a life expectancy of ≥3 months or have had surgery ≥2 months before enrolment (presumably, they also had to give informed consent and speak Italian).	• Controls came from the same cancer centres, with the same eligibility. The intention was to match two controls for each case, using study centre, age, gender, cancer site, histology, and stage.

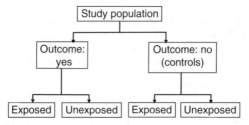

Figure 6.1 General design of a case–control study. 'Outcome' could be any pre-defined event, such as a disorder, death, or other characteristic (e.g. did or did not stop smoking).

Box 6.2 Example of a case–control study where the outcome measure was based on 'counting people' [5]

Objective: To examine whether aspects of sleeping environment increase the risk of SIDS.

Study participants: Mothers of 195 babies who died from SIDS, and 780 controls (mothers of babies who did not die), matched for age and geographical location.

Location: Three health service regions within the UK.

Design: Cases (mothers of babies who died from SIDS) and controls (mothers of babies who did not die). A research team member visited the mother of a SIDS case within 5 days of the death for a face-to-face interview, after informed consent was granted. A second face-to-face interview took place a few days later, when the mother was asked to complete a structured questionnaire. The same questionnaire was given to the control mothers by the researcher (in person), and this visit occurred within a week of the death of the matched case. The questionnaire contained >600 items (including demographic and social characteristics, lifestyle habits, and details about the sleeping environment of the baby when put to bed for the last time).

Exposure: The exposures of interest were factors associated with how the baby was put to bed, with a focus on sleeping position.

Outcome measure: Presence or absence of SIDS. Cases were diagnosed through routine clinical practice.

Results: Results are in Tables 6.2 and 6.3.

Authors' conclusions: Prone (lying face down) and side sleeping positions, covers of the head, and sharing the bed with parents were all important risk factors for SIDS, which could be avoided through education of parents and healthcare professionals.

---

systems, death certificates, or perhaps found through surveys of the general population. Electronic databases are an efficient method of finding cases because it might also be possible to apply some key eligibility criteria at the outset, before contacting potential participants (saving time).

When considering a disorder, the cases could either be newly diagnosed or have had the disorder for some time; the difference between the two matters when considering the time sequence feature for assessing causality (see Box 2.6). For newly diagnosed cases, asking about past exposures usually

Box 6.3 Example of a case–control study where the outcome measure was based on 'taking measurements on people' [6]

Objective: To examine whether head circumference differs between people with and without Alzheimer's disease.

Study participants: 592 patients diagnosed with Alzheimer's disease (cases) and 459 people without dementia (controls).

Location: A single specialist Alzheimer's research centre in the US.

Design: All cases and controls came from the single centre. The controls were volunteers participating in another research study. Research nurses measured head circumference in all participants. Other data were collected from hospital records, and baseline questionnaires.

Exposure: Head circumference, measured in a systematic and pre-defined way – from the glabella to the occipital protuberance, by holding the tape measure taut and avoiding the inclusion of the scalp hair, ears, and any other features that could get in the way.

Outcome measure: Presence or absence of Alzheimer's disease. Cases were diagnosed by neurologists through routine clinical practice, using standard criteria recommended by the US Department of Health and Human Services Task Force on Alzheimer's Disease.

Results: The results are presented in Tables 6.5 and 6.6.

Authors' conclusions: There was a small difference in head circumference between people with and without Alzheimer's disease, but this disappeared when allowing for other factors.

Box 6.4 Example of a case–control study where the outcome measure was based on time-to-event data [7]

Objective: To examine whether the presence of VTE was associated with survival among patients with cancer.

Study participants: 237 cancer patients with VTE (cases) and 339 without VTE (controls) were included. An attempt was made to match for several factors.

Location: 51 cancer centres across Italy.

Design: The study finished recruiting in December 2009, but it was not stated when it started. Cases and controls came from the same cancer centres. Data were extracted from patient records or obtained from patients during their routine assessments (demographic and clinical characteristics, and features of the cancer).

Exposure: The presence (exposed) or absence (unexposed) of VTE diagnosed during routine clinical practice. The VTE status was not determined for controls.

Outcome measure: Overall survival (time until death or date of last follow-up) was assessed during routine clinic assessments.

Results: Figure 6.4 shows the main results.

Authors' conclusions: Cancer patients with VTE were more likely to die early than those without VTE.

guarantees that the exposure occurred before the disorder; but this cannot be assumed for participants with existing disease.

Researchers may also consider whether cases need to be free from other disorders (comorbidities).

Selecting the controls

A difficult design aspect is deciding who should be controls and how to select them [8], and this will also depend on resources and time available for the study. Box 6.5 shows common sources of controls. It is important that controls are representative of the population of interest and that they have similar characteristics to the cases, with the exception of the exposure. If there really is no association between the exposure and outcome, the proportion of controls that is exposed should be the same as that for cases. Care must be taken to avoid choosing controls that lead to a bias, which over- or underestimates the association.

Approaching participants who could become controls may be straightforward if using a well-defined list (hospital/clinic list), or nominations directly from the case (family member or friend). However, using general population sources (e.g. register of residents or neighbour controls) requires careful planning. A random sample is needed because it would be impractical and unnecessary to include everyone. There are various methods of random sampling, ranging from simple random selection, to random sampling that targets groups of people with certain characteristics. **Random digit dialling,** which requires the person to have a telephone, also involves problems with trying to distinguish residential from business numbers, and people who do not pick up when they do not recognise the researchers' telephone number (caller display on digital systems). Many numbers may need to be dialled, just to get one eligible study participant.

Box 6.1 illustrates the various ways in which controls could be selected (using the three examples covered in this chapter). The study of head circumference and Alzheimer's disease used participants from another ongoing study, conducted at the same institution, from which the cases were identified. This is acceptable as long as the controls are considered to be appropriate comparators, that is, they have similar characteristics (which may not always be true if the other study has particular eligibility criteria).

Using hospital/clinic patients as controls is common. Access to these patients is easier than access to the general population, and several patient characteristics (e.g. age, gender, and ethnic origin) should already be available from the hospital database, and so can be used as selection or eligibility criteria. The key difference between these participants and those from the general population is that they all have a disorder, and it is therefore important to ensure that the disorder they have is not associated with the exposure of interest, because this is likely to dilute or mask the association between the disorder being investigated and the exposure.

For example, consider a case–control study to examine the relationship between smoking and lung cancer (Table 6.1). Cases would be patients diagnosed with lung cancer, but suppose the controls were people with heart disease.

Box 6.5 Sources of controls for a case–control study

Population based

Register of people at one or more family physician clinics (i.e. from general practice)	• If the cases have also been selected from this source, these controls could be considered representative of the population from which the cases come. An advantage is that the register (sampling frame) should contain basic characteristics, such as age and gender, which could be applied as eligibility criteria.
Local/national register of residents	• These should be representative of the general population; however, many people would need to be approached in order to achieve the target controls, as many decline to participate. • People who decline could differ from those who do, creating a potential bias.
Neighbourhood controls (people who reside close to the case)	• Could be comparable to cases in terms of socio-economic status, but this approach would require access to a local register of residents or physically visiting the residence of each case and knocking on doors. • Potential bias could arise if contact is attempted during the day, when many people are out.

Other sources

Hospital or clinic patients	• A common source of controls, especially when the cases come from the same institution(s). Eligibility criteria could be applied to the list (details of age, gender, etc should be available). But controls could have other disorders (from the one of interest) and so may be unrepresentative of the population from which the cases come.
Family members of the case	• Asking the case to nominate a close family member could produce a control group comparable to the cases (similar social and lifestyle habits, and genes). It is also relatively easy to obtain controls. However, overmatching could occur for some exposures (habits of family members are likely to be correlated). • Genetic studies may require unrelated controls.
Friends of the case	• Similar potential aspects as family members, except for the genetic similarity.
Volunteers	• Researchers could use themselves or colleagues but they are unlikely to be comparable to the cases. Although easy to obtain it may not be scientifically sound. Possible exceptions could be investigating exposures that are biochemical/biological, which are not influenced by social or demographic characteristics.

Table 6.1 How selecting controls that have similar characteristics, and hence exposure (here smoking) status, to cases can underestimate the association, than if using general population controls.

	Cases with lung cancer	Hospital controls with heart disease	General population controls
	N = 100	N = 400	N = 1000
% of smokers	80	40	20
Risk ratio of smoking*	1	2	4

*% cases ÷ % controls.

If people with heart disease had the same smoking prevalence as the general population, there would be no problem (80/20=4), but if a larger proportion of the heart disease controls smoked, this would underestimate the association between smoking and lung cancer (80/40=2).

It is also possible to identify controls that overestimate an association. For example, if examining the relationship between the risk of colorectal cancer and using non-steroidal anti-inflammatory drugs (NSAIDs) [8], cases could come from a cancer clinic. If controls were selected from gastrointestinal clinics, they would presumably include a proportion with stomach ulcers, who would usually have been told to avoid NSAIDs. Because the proportion exposed to NSAIDs would be lower in this group than in the general population, the association between colorectal cancer and NSAIDs would be overestimated.

There may be situations where hospital controls could be a better match to cases than general population controls (see example in Box 6.4).

Should the controls be matched to cases?
The concept of attempting to 'make everything the same' between the exposed and unexposed group (see page 5), with the exception of the exposure status itself, was presented. Randomised clinical trials can achieve this at the design stage. For most observational studies, differences in potential confounding factors can only be allowed (adjusted) for at the end of the study, during the statistical analysis. However, in a case–control study, the situation can be somewhat different. Cases and controls are selected on the basis of their disease status, and the purpose is to compare the exposure status between them. Therefore, it is expected that the cases (with a disorder) and controls (without) would have different characteristics. Instead of trying to make the exposed and unexposed groups 'the same', researchers can attempt to achieve this with the cases and controls (**matching**). Interest is only in a specified exposure factor, which should be different between cases and controls if it has a real association with the outcome measure (i.e. the disease status).

A **matched case–control study** attempts to 'make everything the same' at the design stage. Researchers specify a few key factors, which are already known or expected to be important confounders. They then select one or more control participants who have the same features for the factors as one of the cases

---

Box 6.6 Approaches to matching in case–control studies

• No matching at all.
• Individual matching: select controls according to specific features of *each case*.
• Frequency matching: select a *group* of controls that generally has similar features to a *group* of cases.

(called **individual matching**). This is the method used by the studies of SIDS and of cancer patients (Box 6.1). In the SIDS study, each control was carefully matched to be as close as possible to each case, using birth date (age) and geographical location. Therefore, the control group should be 'the same' as the cases, in terms of age and location, and any difference in the exposure status cannot be due to these two factors. There are several approaches to matching (Box 6.6). Matched controls can only be achieved if the matching factors are available from the sampling frame (or other source). If matching factors are not available, it might be possible to match by using initial information obtained from responders.

The simplest approach is not to match at all, which is commonly done. If there were no matching, an extreme observation could be that all the SIDS cases were aged <6 months old, and all the controls >12 months. It would then be impossible to separate out the effect of age from the disease status. The study of head circumference (Box 6.3) had no matching at all. In some cases the sampling frame for the controls is known to be generally similar to that for cases, so not having direct matching might be acceptable.

It is important in planning a study to specify how close the matching should be. For example, using exact age is ideal, but it might be difficult to get several controls with the same age as a case. The degree of matching could be relaxed, for example, using age within ±6 or 12 months, which is easier to do, although the greater the allowance, the more different the controls could become.

Determining the number of matching factors depends on the size of the sampling frame for controls. If there are many factors (e.g. ≥10) it will be difficult to find enough matched controls to choose from the sampling frame, unless the list contains a large number of individuals. This was the case for the study in Box 6.4 (and Box 6.1), which attempted to match for six factors. The authors encountered great difficulty in finding suitable matched controls. Using between one and four matching factors would generally be reasonable. The researchers should agree the most important ones. There is a potential for **overmatching**, where the controls selected are so similar to cases that the exposure factor is also similar,[#] and so the association either no longer exists or is diluted. This can arise when one or more of the matching (confounding) factors lies on the same biological/causal pathway as the exposure of interest.

[#]This is the only factor that we want to be different between cases and controls, if the aim is to show an association between the exposure and outcome measure (e.g. disease status).

An alternative to individual matching is **frequency matching**. Instead of finding controls for *each* case, based on one or more factors, a *group* of controls is found that is generally similar to the group of cases. For example, suppose two matching factors are age and smoking status. If, among 120 cases, 20% are aged 50–59 and they smoke, a similar proportion is randomly selected from controls with the same characteristics.

The physical act of selecting matched controls can be quite awkward to deal with, and so often requires the help of an IT programmer to write coding to do this electronically. Some researchers have the two lists (cases and controls) in front of them on paper, and manually select the controls, but this can be laborious and prone to error (especially with several matching factors). The process should ensure that a control is not selected for two or more cases, when using individual matching.

6.3 Measuring variables, exposures, and outcomes

In a case–control study, because the disease status of the cases and controls are known from the outset, the following are key considerations when measuring exposures and other factors (the same principles covered in Section 5.3):
- Standard, established, or generally accepted criteria should be used for diagnosing the cases.
- The exposures should always be assessed using the same methods for both cases and controls, to avoid bias.
- Where applicable (and possible), exposures should be assessed by researchers who do not know the case/control status of the participant (i.e. they are blind to this). If this is not possible, the main study hypotheses should be kept from those collecting data, particularly if they are to conduct direct interviews with the participants. This may be less of an issue if the data have already been recorded in, for example, hospital/medical records, when measures were taken before the current project was planned.
- Consideration could be given to whether controls should have baseline assessments to confirm that they do not have the disorder of interest (though sometimes this is not possible or feasible).

6.4 Collecting the data

As with other observational studies, data from case–control studies can be collected using a variety of sources (see Box 1.9)

Some case–control studies also involve collecting data from a proxy or surrogate, who could be a relative, next of kin, or possibly a friend. This is done when the case is unavailable, for example, has died or is unfit or unable to be interviewed or complete questionnaires.

As with cross-sectional studies, researchers on case–control studies should specify clearly, at the start, which information they require, because there is usually only one attempt to obtain this from the study participants or their proxy.

6.5 Sample size

All sample size estimations are guesses. There is nothing precise or accurate about them. Even with what appears to be reliable information used in the estimation, the achieved study size could still be too big or too small.

The number of 'events' (disorder, death, or other defined occurrence) matters greatly, in that it influences the reliability of the statistical analyses (see Box 3.8). A major advantage of a case–control study is that the researchers can choose the number of events (cases). Another key consideration is the number of controls. Some researchers believe that the more controls they include, the better, but while having up to four controls per case is appropriate, more than four does not significantly improve the reliability of the statistical analyses.

In the SIDS study in Boxes 6.1 and 6.2, four controls per case were chosen. With 196 cases, a target of 780 controls (4×196) was specified and achieved. In some studies, selected controls may be found subsequently to have missing key information, and so may be excluded from the statistical analysis. Therefore, although researchers specify the target number of controls per case, the number actually recruited and analysed may be less. The study on Alzheimer's disease did not specify a target number of controls, because the size of this group was already fixed (they came from an ongoing study). In this situation, there were more cases than controls (592 vs. 459), which is generally not a problem, as long as the control group is sufficiently large.

Information needed for sample size estimation when examining associations

When case–control studies aim to examine the effect of a single exposure factor on a single outcome measure (e.g. disorder), several pieces of information are needed for the sample size calculation (Figure 6.2). Items such as the percentage of controls expected to be classified as exposed should ideally come from prior information.

The magnitude of the effect size (odds ratio OR) could be based on previous knowledge or one that is judged to be associated with a minimum clinically important effect. The smaller the expected effect size, the larger the study that is required. In the example in Figure 6.2, the OR is 2.0 (a reasonably large effect), and this requires 400 participants (100 cases and 300 controls). If the OR were 1.5, the study size would greatly increase, to 1200 participants (300 cases and 900 controls). Choosing a sample size that seems feasible in a certain time frame and *then* specifying the effect size is an inappropriate approach, because the effect size could be quite different in reality from what was expected. The sample size estimate only reflects the contributing assumptions. If the assumptions are unrealistic, the size of the study will be too small or too large.

There are several methods available to calculate the sample size from statistical packages and software [9, 10], including those freely available for observational studies [11].

When the outcome measure is based on 'counting people' or time-to-event data (both use risk), the number of events is often more important than the total

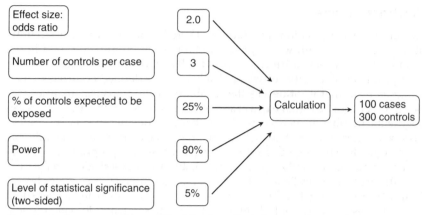

Sample size increases with any of the following: effect size gets closer to the no, effect value, or % of controls exposed reduces.

Figure 6.2 Information required for a sample size estimation for case–control studies in which the effect size is an OR.

number of participants in the study. For 'taking measurements on people', the standard deviation of the endpoint will influence study size (little variability between participants requires a smaller study).

In Figure 6.2, the **level of statistical significance** is the chance of finding an effect when in reality one does not exist, so the conclusion of the study would be wrong. It is essentially an error rate, and is often set at 5% (0.05). The results will be determined to be statistically significant at this level, which is generally regarded to be sufficiently low before making conclusions about the association. A lower error rate (1%) may be used, which increases sample size.

Power can be interpreted as the chance of finding an effect size of the magnitude specified, if it really exists. Most studies use a high power, such as 80 or 90%. Using the example in Figure 6.2, if the <u>true</u> OR is at least 2.0, a study size of 400 participants should mean that there is an 80% chance of finding this size of effect or greater and that it would be statistically significant at the 5% level. Increasing power will increase the sample size.

The method of sample size calculation depends on the type of outcome measure and effect size used:

- Counting people (OR)
- Taking measurements on people (mean difference)
- Time-to-event data (hazard ratio)

When there are several exposures to examine, and no one particular exposure has been designated as the item of interest, estimating sample size is complex. An estimate could be made for each factor, and a simple approach would be to then take the largest sample size. However, if this size is unfeasible, it may be appropriate to attempt to reduce the number of exposures, and to identify two or three key factors, for which sample sizes could then be examined. If the researchers plan to include all the factors in a multivariable regression analysis, at least 10 events (cases) would be required [12]; this would not involve the concept of statistical power.

6.6 Analysing data and interpreting results

Prevalence and incidence are useful ways of measuring disease occurrence (see Box 2.2). Prevalence can be estimated from cross-sectional studies, and incidence from cohort studies; however, case–control studies include a specified number of cases and controls (determined by the researchers), so it is not possible to obtain either prevalence or incidence.

Continuous exposure variables can be divided into groups of similar size, such as tertiles or quartiles (see page 76). However, rather than combining cases and controls, just using the controls (i.e. those without the disorder of interest) should give a clearer association between the exposure and outcome. If there is a relationship, the cases (those with the disorder) should tend to have values at one end of the distribution. Using all the study participants to define the cut-off points will yield an artificial ratio of cases to controls (i.e. chosen by the researchers), and because this does not reflect the actual incidence, the cut-off points could dilute or mask an association. Also, if using only controls to define the cut-off points, the group should be more homogenous.

A table showing the key (baseline) characteristics in cases and controls separately, is useful to see how comparable they are.

6.7 Outcome measures based on 'counting people' endpoints: Sudden infant death syndrome and sleeping factors (Box 6.2)

Measuring variables, exposures, and outcomes

The participants in this study were the mother–baby *pair*. The outcome measure related to the health of the baby, while the data on exposures were reported by the mother, and based on her characteristics, the home environment, and the baby's sleeping environment.

There were many exposures (risk factors) in this study, with a focus on how babies were put to bed, particularly sleeping position. The cases (specifically mothers) had to remember several details about the last night the baby was alive, as well as much information about the living environment and her own characteristics. The questionnaire had over 600 items, completed by the mother while the researcher was present. Even a factor like 'sleeping position' (back, side, or face down), which initially appears straightforward, requires thought: there is the position in which the mother put the baby to bed, and the position in which the baby was found after death.

A common potential problem in case–control studies is **recall bias** (see Box 1.6). Because the case has suffered a health-related event, they might be more likely to recall past information more accurately, or possibly over-report exposure status, than controls, who have not had any such event triggered. However, it is also possible in this situation that some mothers might not be able to report information with sufficient accuracy, due to the stressful nature of the topic (the baby would only have died a few days before the interview).

The outcome measure was the occurrence of SIDS, which was diagnosed through routine clinical practice. The control group was babies who were alive.

Analysing data and interpreting results

In a study such as this, in which many variables (>600) were measured performing numerous analyses may lead to a loss of focus on the main exposures of interest. Sleeping position (i.e. whether the baby was put to bed on the front, back, or side) had already been known to be associated with SIDS. This study aimed to confirm the finding, and to also find other potential risk factors. When planning this study, the researchers did not have a specific exposure in mind. Here, it is essential that multivariable statistical analyses are used (see page 77). An exposure of interest in one analysis would be a potential confounding factor in another, and the simultaneous effect of all the factors on the risk of SIDS needs to be examined.

The outcome measure (chance of having a baby with SIDS) was analysed using a **logistic regression** (see page 69). Matching was used to select controls, and this was taken into account in the analyses using **conditional logistic regression** for matched case–control studies. Essentially, the data were analysed within each matched set, which is not the same as adding the matching variables as cofactors to the regression model.

What are the main results?

Table 6.2 is typical for a case–control study. Sometimes, the reference group, which we call **unexposed**, is obvious, for example, never-smoker in a study of cancer and cigarette smoking. In the SIDS study, the reference group was chosen as the 'back' sleeping position, probably because this was already recommended as public health policy at the time.

Table 6.2 Summary table showing all three exposure groups and the odds ratios (ORs) taking into account the matching factors between the cases and controls.

Sleeping position (when put to bed)	Case (baby died from SIDS)	Control (baby alive)	ORs	
			Allowing for the matching factors?	
			No*	Yes**
Back#	82	509	1.0	1.0
Side	76	241	1.96	2.01
Front (face down)	30	24	7.76	9.58

*Can be calculated by hand (e.g. for front vs. back) as follows:
  Odds of SIDS in the exposed group: 30/24 = 1.25.
  Odds of SIDS in the unexposed group: 82/509 = 0.161.
  OR = 1.25/0.161 = 7.76.
**Calculated using a conditional logistic regression.
#Chosen to be the reference group.

The aim is to compare the risk of SIDS between the exposed and unexposed groups, to produce a **relative risk** (see Chapter 3, page 48). However, risk cannot be calculated in a case–control study because the number of cases and controls is artificial, so we cannot obtain either a correct numerator or denominator for risk. Instead, the **odds** of having a baby with SIDS is obtained (Table 6.2) in each exposure group, from which the **OR** can be calculated. Because SIDS is quite uncommon (about 1 in 500 births in the UK in the 1980s), the OR should be a good estimate of the relative risk (see Table 3.2). In the example, it is 7.76, meaning that if the baby were put to bed on its front, it was almost eight times more likely to die from SIDS than a baby on its back. This is a very large effect.

This is a crude OR (ignoring matching), but it is common practice to report the estimate after allowing for the matching factors (here, age and geographical location) using a conditional logistic regression (Table 6.2). Babies put to bed on their sides had twice the risk of SIDS compared with those put down on their backs, and the risk was more than 9 times higher for those on their front. The results in Table 6.2 focus on the sleeping position of the baby and confirm the findings and conclusions from previous studies.

Table 6.3 shows the association between SIDS and several factors of interest. Although the first column is labelled 'univariable (unadjusted)', the ORs have already allowed for the matching factors (age and geographical location). The

Table 6.3 Factors associated with the sleeping environment.

	Univariable odds ratio (unadjusted)	Multivariable (adjusted) odds ratio
Sleeping position:		
Front (prone)	9.58 (4.86–18.87)	9 (2.84–28.47)
Side sleeping	2.01 (1.38–2.93)	1.84 (1.02–3.31)
Found with covers over head	18.93 (8.05–44.48)	21.58 (6.21–74.99)
Bedding:		
6–9 togs**	1.5 (0.99–2.26)	0.89 (0.45–1.76)
≥10 togs**	3.38 (1.94–5.87)	0.94 (0.31–2.83)
Wearing hat	p = 0.015*	4.13 (0.22–77.89)
Heating on all night	2.14 (1.30–3.50)	2.37 (0.96–5.84)
Mothers who ever breastfed	0.5 (0.35–0.71)	1.06 (0.57–1.98)
Shared bed with parents	4.12 (2.30–7.40)	4.36 (1.59–11.95)
Used dummy (pacifier)	0.59 (0.42–0.84)	0.38 (0.21–0.70)
Used duvet	2.82 (1.95–4.08)	1.72 (0.90–3.30)
Loose bed covering	1.92 (1.35–2.73)	1.07 (0.61–1.89)

*Adjusted for maternal age, parity, gestation, birthweight, whether family received income supplement, exposure to tobacco smoke, and the sleeping factors in the table that remained statistically significant after adjustment.
*OR not reliable because of small numbers (p-value from Fisher's exact test).
**'Tog' is a measure of the warmth (thickness) of the bedding/duvet.
The reference (comparison) group for each factor is not shown in the table, to avoid having multiple rows with OR 1.0. It is the opposite of what is shown for all factors, for example, the reference for 'mothers who ever breastfed,' is 'mothers who never breastfed,' except for sleeping position (reference is 'back' and for bedding '<6 togs').

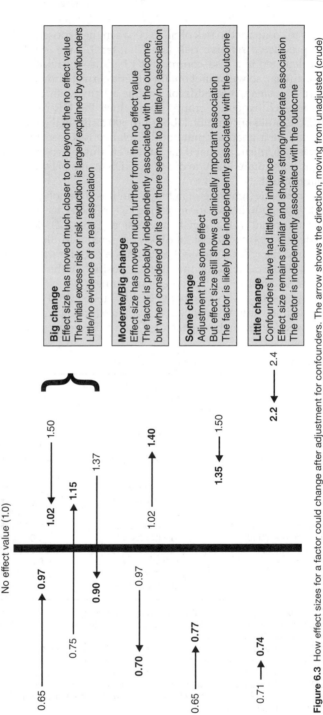

Relative risk, odds ratio, or hazard ratio
No effect value (1.0)

Big change
Effect size has moved much closer to or beyond the no effect value
The initial excess risk or risk reduction is largely explained by confounders
Little/no evidence of a real association

Moderate/Big change
Effect size has moved much further from the no effect value
The factor is probably independently associated with the outcome, but when considered on its own there seems to be little/no association

Some change
Adjustment has some effect
But effect size still shows a clinically important association
The factor is likely to be independently associated with the outcome

Little change
Confounders have had little/no influence
Effect size remains similar and shows strong/moderate association
The factor is independently associated with the outcome

Figure 6.3 How effect sizes for a factor could change after adjustment for confounders. The arrow shows the direction, moving from unadjusted (crude) estimate to adjusted (shown as bold). The 95% CIs also need to be interpreted, in terms of whether they include the no effect value or not.

reason for this labelling is that the matching factors have not been treated in the same way as the other variables in the regression model.

Table 6.3 is useful because it shows the association between each exposure factor individually and also when adjusted for other factors. Because there is interest in whether the size of the effect changes, and whether it moves closer to the no effect value, both unadjusted and adjusted effect sizes should be reported (Figure 6.3).

Box 6.7 is an interpretation of the results in Table 6.3. ORs above 1.0 indicate that the risk of SIDS increased compared with the reference group, and those below 1.0 indicate a protective effect (risk decreased). The more extreme the value, the stronger the risk factor (Figure 3.1). Those with the strongest association are, in order of magnitude, as follows: 'found with covers over head' (OR 21.58), 'sleeping on front' (OR 9), 'sharing bed with parents' (OR 4.36), and 'using dummy/pacifier' (OR 0.38#). Because these effects remained similar and statistically significant after adjustment, they could be referred to as **independent risk factors**, and this is one of the features for causality (Box 2.6).

Factors that initially appeared to have a clear association with the risk of SIDS (e.g. bedding tog ≥10, mothers who breastfed, and loose bed covering), had adjusted ORs close to 1.0, indicating that each of these associations was actually due to the other factors in the table, and not the exposure factor itself. It is difficult to ascertain which factors made the associations disappear, especially when there are many to consider and the relationship between them might be complex. What is important is that they were taken into account.

What could the true effect be, given that the study was conducted on a sample of people?

Table 6.3 shows the 95% CI for all the factors. Several intervals are wide, suggesting that the number of babies in the relevant 'exposed' group may not have been large (thus contributing to make the standard error larger). For example, the interval for the strongest risk factor (found with covers over head) is 6.21–74.99. Despite this being very wide, even the lower limit (the expected conservative estimate of the true effect) is 6.21, which is still a large effect.

As shown in Box 6.7, if the 95% CI includes the no effect value after adjustment for other factors, it is possible that the true OR could be 1.0, indicating no association. Some factors (bedding tog ≥10, mothers who breastfed, and loose bed covering) had unadjusted 95% CIs that excluded 1.0, but after adjustment they easily included 1.0. One possible exception was 'heating on all night', for which the adjusted CI just overlapped 1.0 (lower limit 0.96), but the point estimate of the OR remained high (2.37). The true OR is more likely to lie around the middle of the interval than at either end (see page 58).

An OR of 0.38 is equivalent to 1/0.38 = 2.63 as an increase in risk, if comparing not using a pacifier with using one.

Box 6.7 Interpretation of selected results from Table 6.3

Factor	Comments (the no effect value is 1.0, indicating no association) (OR = odds ratio)	Is it an independent risk factor (i.e. the adjusted OR remains away from 1.0 and statistically significant)*?
Sleeping position (side or front)	Front sleeping has the strongest effect (10-fold increase in risk); side sleeping has about a twofold increase. These effects remains largely the same after adjustment for other factors	Yes
Found with covers over head	The strongest risk factor in the table (most extreme value away from 1.0). There is a 21-fold increase in risk; this is very large	Yes
Bedding (tog value)	On its own, a high tog value looks like a risk factor (3.38-fold increase in risk for ≥10 togs), but after adjustment, the OR is close to 1.0	No
Heating on all night	The unadjusted OR indicates a doubling in risk, and the adjusted estimates remain similar or higher	Possibly; the 95% CI adjusted for all factors just includes 1.0 (lower limit 0.96)
Mothers who ever breastfed	Looks like a strong *protective* effect, when considered on its own; the risk of SIDS is halved (OR 0.5). But after adjustment, there is hardly any effect, OR close to 1.0	No
Used dummy (pacifier)	Looks like a strong protective effect, when considered on its own; the risk of SIDS is almost halved (OR 0.59). After adjustment, the effect is slightly stronger	Yes

* 95% CI excludes 1.0

Box 6.8 Estimating a p-value using an odds ratio (OR), relative risk or hazard ratio, and its 95% CI

Effect sizes based on ratios are usually analysed on a $\log_e$ scale:

95% confidence limit $= \log_e(\text{OR}) \pm 1.96 \times$ standard error

$\log_e(\text{upper 95% confidence limit}) = \log_e(\text{OR}) + 1.96 \times$ standard error

The OR for sleeping on the side is 1.84, with 95% CI 1.02–3.31:

$\log_e(3.31) = \log_e(1.84) + 1.96 \times$ standard error

$$\text{Standard error} = \frac{\log_e(3.31) - \log_e(1.84)}{1.96} = 0.300$$

We can then see how far the OR of 1.84 is from the no effect value, in standard errors:

$$\frac{\log_e(1.84) - \log_e(1.0)}{0.300} = 2.03 \left(\text{referred to as a z-score, or standard Normal score} \right)$$

Using Normal (Gaussian) tables, a z-score of 2.03 is associated with a two-sided p-value of 0.04. The higher the z-value, the smaller the p-value below 0.05:

If z-score (ignoring sign) is	Two-tailed p-value is
> 1.96	< 0.05
> 2.57	< 0.01
> 3.29	< 0.001
> 3.89	< 0.0001

Could the observed result be a chance finding in this particular study?
No p-values were published, but Figure 3.7 could be used to determine whether the p-value is above or below 0.05, given the location of the 95% CI in relation to the no effect value. The size of the p-value can also be estimated using the approach outlined in Box 6.8, which should be reasonably close to that obtained directly from the logistic regression analysis (Table 6.4).

The estimated p-values for several factors are very small, providing good evidence for each association (Table 6.4). For example, the OR for 'covers over head' is very large (21.58). The p-value of <0.0001 tells us that an effect as large as this (or more extreme) could be due to chance, if there really were no effect, but we would only expect to see this in fewer than 1 in 10,000 similarly sized studies. As this is highly unlikely to occur, it is probable that the effect is real. The p-value for breastfeeding based on the unadjusted OR of 0.50 is 0.0001 (highly statistically significant), but when adjusted it changes to 0.85, showing the importance of allowing for potential confounding factors, to avoid making incorrect conclusions.

Table 6.4 Estimated p-values for selected adjusted odds ratio in the 'multivariable' column of Table 6.3 (using Box 6.8).

Risk factor	OR	Estimated p-value
Sleeping on front	9	0.0002
Sleeping on side	1.84	0.04
Found with covers over head	21.58	<0.0001
Heating on all night	2.37	0.06
Mother who ever breastfed	1.06	0.85
Using dummy/pacifier	0.38	0.002

Box 6.9 Consideration of causality in relation to the exposure 'putting babies to bed on their front' (see Box 2.6)

Feature	Comments
Does exposure come before the outcome?	Technically yes, in this case, because the baby died so any exposure must have preceded it. But it is not possible to confirm that the recorded sleeping position was the one <u>directly</u> before the death in the study
Is the association strong and statistically significant after adjustment for confounders?	Yes
Does risk increase with increasing exposure?	Not applicable (either baby is put to sleep on the front or not)
Does risk decrease if the exposure is removed?	Cannot ascertain from this study. But after campaigns began informing mothers not to put babies to bed on their fronts, the birth prevalence of SIDS decreased dramatically
Is there supporting evidence from other studies?	Yes; good evidence from several other independent studies
Is there biological plausibility	Yes; placing babies on their front is likely to interfere with their breathing

How good is the evidence?

This is a relatively large study (195 cases), given that SIDS was uncommon. A further strength was the amount of information collected, which consequently allowed for a comprehensive statistical analysis, adjusting for many known potential confounders. This meant that exposures (risk factors) with extreme ORs that were highly statistically significant after adjustment were likely to be independent risk factors. The main limitation was recall bias (as in many case–control studies): whether the mothers of babies with SIDS were more likely to remember accurately how their baby was put to bed than the control mothers. However, even if this bias existed to some extent, it is unlikely to explain such large effect sizes.

It is appropriate to consider whether the associations found were likely to be causal (Box 2.6). For sleeping on the front, a series of observations could be made in relation to the features for causality (see Box 6.9), and from these it is therefore likely that the association between sleeping position and risk of SIDS is causal.

The final step is determining how to use the study findings, and whether they should influence public health policy and education. Given that the factors found to have strong associations were ones that can be changed by parents, it would be appropriate to make recommendations for future parents.

6.8 Measures based on 'taking measurements on people' endpoints: Alzheimer's disease and head circumference (Box 6.3)

Measuring variables, exposures, and outcomes

In other chapters, examples are given where the endpoint (outcome) was based on 'taking measurements on people' (continuous measure), but this concept does not readily apply to case–control studies, because a continuous measure in itself is not a disorder. However, researchers could divide it into two or more groups, and select participants on this basis. For example, cases could be individuals with high blood pressure (>140 mmHg systolic and >90 diastolic), and controls could have values within the normal range. Then the outcome is the same as 'counting people' endpoints.

In Box 6.3, the exposure was head circumference, measured by registered research nurses, using the same standard approach for both cases and controls. This was essential to avoid any bias, which could arise if the nurses tended to record larger head circumferences for the cases than the controls, so that any observed difference in this measurement between cases and controls was due to the nurse, and not the disease status.

The research nurses measuring head circumference in this study would have known the disease status of the participants because they came from known different sources. The question is whether this matters here. Head circumference was measured routinely as part of the diagnosis for cases since 1992, and for the controls it was probably one of several measurements obtained for the research study in which they were already enrolled. Therefore, the research nurses may not have been aware of the future plan to look at the specific association between head circumference and Alzheimer's disease, which was conducted in 2005/2006. Even so, the potential for bias cannot be excluded completely.

The outcome measure (Alzheimer's disease) was assessed by neurologists through routine clinical practice, using standard criteria recommended by the US Department of Health and Human Services Task Force on Alzheimer's Disease.

Analysing data and interpreting results

This study was analysed using a **linear regression** (see Chapter 4). The outcome measure (having Alzheimer's disease) was treated as a cofactor (exposure) in the regression model, while the exposure (head circumference) was treated as the endpoint (which is a continuous measurement). However, this does not really matter when interpreting the findings, because in these types of case–control studies, interest is in the association, rather than which factor preceded which (in order to consider causality).

What are the main results?

Table 6.5 compares head circumference, age and education between the cases and controls. Results are presented according to sex because head circumference is known to be larger among males (confirmed in the table). In both sexes, the cases are older than controls, and they have had fewer years of education, providing evidence that these two factors are associated with the presence of Alzheimer's disease, making them potential confounders.

The table also shows that head circumference is smaller among cases than controls for both sexes. The effect size is a **mean difference**: head circumference is 0.58 cm smaller among males, and 0.32 cm smaller among females. Although these effect sizes indicate an association between head circumference and the presence of Alzheimer's disease, they are quite small when considered in relation to a typical total head circumference of 55–58 cm.

The multivariable linear regression results are shown in Table 6.6. When the factor is a continuous measure (age and years of education), the effect size is a **regression coefficient** (i.e. how much does head circumference change when the factor increases by one unit). For factors with two levels, that is, sex (males or females), family relative with dementia (yes or no), and Alzheimer's disease (yes or no), the effect size is simply the mean difference[#] in head circumference between the levels. Box 6.10 shows the interpretation of the results.

All of the effect sizes have been adjusted for all the other factors included in the regression. There is no longer a difference between cases and controls: the mean difference in head circumference has changed from −0.58 (males) and −0.32 cm (females) to a small value −0.043 cm.

What could the true effect be, given that the study was conducted on a sample of people?

Table 6.5 shows that the 95% CI for the unadjusted mean differences were relatively narrow: 0.22–0.94 for males and 0.09–0.55 for females. Narrow intervals, associated with small standard errors, are due to the relatively moderate sample sizes, but also the small standard deviations. Even the upper estimates of the mean difference are not large: 0.94 (males) and 0.55 cm (females). The important result is the adjusted mean difference (Table 6.6), for which the 95% CI (−0.289 to +0.203) easily overlaps the no effect value of zero, indicating that the true difference could be zero (no association between head circumference and presence of Alzheimer's disease).

[#] The regression coefficient is the same as a mean difference.

Table 6.5 Head circumference and two other potential confounding factors according to disease status. The table shows the mean values (standard deviations in brackets).

	Males			Females		
	Cases	Controls	Difference	Cases	Controls	Difference
	N = 164	N = 161		N = 428	N = 298	
Head circumference (cm)	57.46 (1.65)	58.04 (1.63)	−0.58	55.14 (1.64)	55.46 (1.46)	−0.32
Age (years)	76.4 (6.7)	71.4 (6.1)	+5.0	78.0 (6.7)	71.2 (7.3)	+6.8
Education (years)	13.0 (7.9)	16.4 (2.5)	−3.4	12.7 (8.0)	15.5 (2.2)	−2.8

For head circumference, the 95% CI and p-values for the difference among males can be calculated to be 0.22–0.94 (p = 0.002); and for females, it is 0.09–0.55 (p = 0.007), using N, means and standard deviations [13].
Cases: Alzheimer's disease, controls: unaffected.

Table 6.6 Results of the multivariable linear regression analysis.

	Regression coefficient (95% CI)	p-value
Alzheimer's disease	−0.043 (−0.289, +0.203)	0.30
Sex	2.38 (2.17, 2.59)	<0.0001
Age at baseline	−0.031 (−0.045, −0.017)	<0.0001
Years of education	0.067 (0.037, 0.097)	0.019
Relative with dementia	0.030 (−0.172, 0.231)	0.30

A negative coefficient indicates that head circumference decreases when the factor increases, and when positive it increases. For sex, the coefficient is the mean among males minus the mean among females. The no effect value is 0.

Could the observed result be a chance finding in this particular study?
The p-values for the unadjusted mean differences (Table 6.5) are surprisingly small (p = 0.002 and 0.007), given the small effect sizes, but again this is partly due to small standard errors. The main p-value comes from Table 6.6, which shows the p-value for the difference in head circumference between cases and controls is 0.30. This indicates that a difference of −0.043 (or more extreme) could be due to chance in 3 out of 10 similar sized studies, providing little evidence for a real effect. There is, however, evidence for an independent association with sex, age and education.

How good is the evidence?
Although this was a reasonably sized study, the unadjusted effect size showed a clinically small effect; but after adjustment for four potential confounders, there was little evidence of an association. One limitation is that Alzheimer's disease is a complex disorder, and there may be unknown (and therefore

---

Box 6.10 Interpretation of the results in Table 6.6

Factor	Comments
Alzheimer's disease	Cases with Alzheimer's disease had a mean head circumference that is 0.043 cm lower than the controls
Sex	The mean difference in head circumference between males and females is +2.38 cm, that is, on average this measure was 2.38 cm larger among males
Age at baseline (years)	As age increased by 1 year, the mean head circumference reduces by 0.031 cm
Education (years)	As the number of years of education increased by 1 year, the mean head circumference increased by 0.067 cm
Relative with dementia	If the participant had a family history of dementia, their head circumference was on average 0.03 cm larger than someone without a history

Effect sizes have been adjusted for the other factors.

---

unmeasured) confounders that, because they were not allowed for, may have masked the association. It is also possible that head size could have been based on imaging to estimate brain volume, which is perhaps a better measure of the exposure, given the hypothesis that having more neurons delay or protect against the disorder.

6.9 Outcome measures based on time-to-event endpoints: Venous thromboembolism (VTE) and survival (Box 6.4)

Measuring variables, exposures, and outcomes
In this example, the controls were deliberately chosen to come from the same target population as the cases, that is, hospital patients. Controls could have been selected from the general population, which might, initially, be considered the best comparator. The choice of control group depends on the research question; in this case, 'Is survival different between cases and either (i) other patients with cancer or (ii) the general population?' As cancer patients and individuals selected from the general population (many of whom are free from cancer) are likely to have many different characteristics, there will therefore be many different potential confounding factors (e.g. age). By choosing cancer patients as controls, the hope would be that they have similar characteristics to the cases, minimising the potential for confounding and maximising the opportunity to 'make everything the same'.

The exposure factor in this study was the presence or absence of a VTE, assessed by the treating clinician, during usual practice. There was a standard

Table 6.7 Selected characteristics of cases and controls.

	Cases (%) N=237	Control (%) N=339	p-value for the difference
Sex			
Males	43.0	41.9	0.78
Females	57.0	58.1	
Age (years)			
<60	29.1	26.3	0.26
60–69	35.4	42.2	
70	35.4	31.6	
Cancer stage			
Locally advanced	6.8	3.8	0.12
Metastatic	93.2	96.2	

definition for this: the VTE had to be diagnosed within 2 months of enrolment to the study using imaging (ultrasound, CT scan, or lung angiography, depending on the location of the VTE). The VTE could be either symptomatic or asymptomatic. However, imaging was not performed among controls to determine their VTE status, so it is plausible that some may have had asymptomatic VTE. Furthermore, it was unclear why some asymptomatic VTE cases had been referred for imaging, and this may also have created some bias.

The outcome measure was straightforward: time to death from any cause, so only the date of death was required during follow-up. Unlike other case–control studies, which only collect data retrospectively, in this example, data were to be collected prospectively. As an alternative, such data could have been obtained from medical records, but there must have been a length of follow-up in the past, for the time-to-event variable to be measured.

Analysing data and interpreting results
The study was analysed using a **Cox regression** (see page 69).

What are the main results?
When cases and controls are selected from very different sampling frames, they are expected to have different characteristics, and a table would show this in the published paper. However, in this study, where the controls also had cancer, there were hardly any differences (Table 6.7).

The outcome measure of time to death among patients with and without VTE and the Kaplan–Meier curves are shown in Figure 6.4. There was a clear difference in overall survival between cases and controls (Figure 6.4a). The unadjusted hazard ratio was 1.79, suggesting that cancer patients with a VTE were 79% more likely to die than cancer patients without VTE. This is a moderate/large effect. The number of patients at risk, given below the figure, shows that there were sufficient patients up to 10 months in each exposure group, making the curves at these points reliable. Even at 12, and possibly 14 months, the number of patients was not negligible. After adjusting for several

(a)

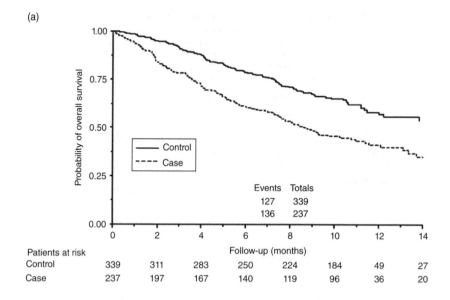

Patients at risk

Control	339	311	283	250	224	184	49	27
Case	237	197	167	140	119	96	36	20

(b)

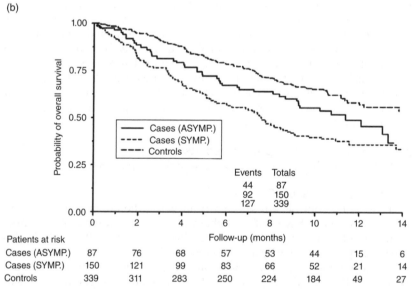

Patients at risk

Cases (ASYMP.)	87	76	68	57	53	44	15	6
Cases (SYMP.)	150	121	99	83	66	52	21	14
Controls	339	311	283	250	224	184	49	27

Figure 6.4 The Kaplan–Meier curves. In (a), the unadjusted hazard ratio is 1.79 (95% CI 1.40–2.28), and the adjusted estimate is 1.55 (95% CI 1.21–2.00). Source: Agnelli et al. 2013 [7]. Reproduced by permission of Springer Science +Business Media.

potential confounders (not specified in the paper, but may have included cancer stage, body mass index, and performance status), the hazard ratio only
reduced to 1.55 (55% increase in risk).

Figure 6.4b is useful because it subdivides the cases into two groups (symptomatic and asymptomatic VTE), showing that those who were symptomatic
had worse survival, as expected, (a *trend* in the Kaplan–Meier curves according to severity of VTE). This kind observation adds further support to a real
association.

What could the true effect be, given that the study was conducted on a sample of people?

The 95% CI for the adjusted hazard ratio was 1.21–2.00, so a conservative estimate
of the true excess risk was 21%, but the true increase in risk could be a doubling.

Could the observed result be a chance finding in this particular study?

No p-value was reported, but using the approach in Box 6.8, it is estimated to
be <0.001. Therefore, an adjusted hazard ratio as large as 1.55 (or more extreme)
is highly unlikely to be due to chance, so there is likely to be a real difference
in survival times between the cases and controls.

How good is the evidence?

The study was relatively large, and the controls were well matched to the
controls. However, the VTE status was not confirmed for controls. If there
had been some undiagnosed patients with VTE among the controls, this
would dilute the hazard ratio. Therefore, it is possible that the adjusted hazard ratio of 1.55 is an underestimate. There is some uncertainty over why
some patients had been referred for assessment of VTE, while others had
not. The reasons (unspecified in the article) could have created a bias, leading to the observed difference in survival between cases and controls. The
important question is whether they could have produced an effect as large
as a hazard ratio of 1.55. Another consideration is whether the VTE cases
were managed differently from controls during follow-up because their status was known at the start. For example, they could have been recalled for
more frequent or different assessments, which might have improved their
survival, but if this did occur it would dilute the hazard ratio.

The study findings and conclusions are consistent with previous studies,
most of which were retrospective. The recommendations from the study
were to find reasons why VTE cancer patients have a worse survival and
also to determine whether preventing VTE could improve survival.

6.10 Key points

- Case–control studies can be an efficient and relatively quick way of examining associations between an exposure and outcome.
- There need to be clear definitions of cases (including methods of diagnosis)
and controls.

- Separate sampling frames are often needed for cases and controls.
- Selecting controls requires much care with regard to where they come from, how they are selected, and whether they should be matched; they should be representative of the population of interest.
- Assessment of cases and controls should be done in the same way to avoid bias.
- Data can come directly from participants, their proxy, or medical records or by flagging them with regional or national databases/registries.
- When examining risk factors and causality, important potential confounders should be allowed for in the statistical analysis.
- The interpretation of effect sizes such as relative risk, OR, mean difference, and hazard ratio (and 95% CIs and p-values) is the same as in other chapters.

References

1. Silman AJ, Macfarlane GJ. Epidemiological Studies: A Practical Guide. Cambridge University Press. Second Edition (2002).
2. Rothman KJ. Epidemiology: An Introduction. Oxford University Press. First Edition (2002).
3. dos Santos Silva I Case-control studies. In: Cancer Epidemiology: Principles and Methods. IARC Press (1999). http://www.iarc.fr/en/publications/pdfs-online/epi/cancerepi/. Accessed 19 May 2014.
4. Schulz KF, Grimes DA. Case-control studies: research in reverse. Lancet 2002;359: 431–4.
5. Fleming PJ, Blair PS, Bacon C, Bensley D, Smith I, Taylor E, et al. Environment of infants during sleep and risk of the sudden infant death syndrome: results of 1993-5 case-control study for confidential inquiry into stillbirths and deaths in infancy. Confidential Enquiry into Stillbirths and Deaths Regional Coordinators and Researchers. BMJ 1996;313(7051):191–5.
6. Espinosa PS, Kryscio RJ, Mendiondo MS, Schmitt FA, Wekstein DR, Markesbery WR, Smith CD. Alzheimer's disease and head circumference. J Alzheimers Dis 2006;9(1): 77–80.
7. Agnelli G, Verso M, Mandalà M, Gallus S, Cimminiello C, Apolone G, et al. A prospective study on survival in cancer patients with and without venous thromboembolism. Intern Emerg Med 2013. PMID: 23943559.
8. Grimes DA, Schulz KF. Compared to what? Finding controls for case-control studies. Lancet 2005;365:1429–33.
9. DuPont WD, Plummer WD. Power and sample size calculation. http://medipe.psu.ac.th/episoft/pssamplesize/. Accessed 19 May 2014.
10. Machin D, Campbell M, Tan SB, Tan SH. Sample Size Tables for Clinical Studies. Wiley-Blackwell. Third Edition (2009).
11. 5. Epi Info, Version 7. US Centers for Disease Control and Prevention. http://wwwn.cdc.gov/epiinfo/7/. Accessed 19 May 2014.
12. Concato J, Peduzzi P, Holford TR, Feinstein AR. Importance of events per independent variable in proportional hazards analysis. I. Background, goals, and general strategy. J Clin Epidemiol 1995;48(12):1495–501.
13. Kirkwood BR, Sterne JAC. Essential Medical Statistics. Blackwell Science. Second Edition (2003).

CHAPTER 7

Cohort studies

7.1 Purpose

Cohort studies are generally considered to be the best type of observational study for evaluating risk factors and causality, and sometimes the natural history of a disorder. Such studies may also be useful in evaluating treatments with large effects, although there may still be uncertainty over the actual size of the effect (if confounding and bias are not adequately allowed for). More details about cohort studies can be found elsewhere [1–4].

7.2 Design

The key difference between a cohort study and the other types of observational studies (i.e. cross-sectional and case–control) is the prospective collection of data. This may occur, to a small extent, in cross-sectional studies, such as in the example in Box 5.5 in which study participants recorded dietary data over a week, but for a cohort study, data need to be collected over a much longer time period (usually months, sometimes years). The ultimate purpose is usually to observe *new* events (e.g. new cases of a specific disorder, changes in habits or lifestyles, or deaths) or how measurements change over time. Figure 7.1 shows the general design of a cohort study.

A common definition of a typical prospective cohort study is that it is based only on people without the disorder of interest at baseline. For example, if examining the association between smoking and cancer, only people free from cancer would be eligible for the study. The participants might be described as 'healthy' individuals, although technically this would be incorrect, because some are likely to have other disorders.[#] However, several cohort studies do not focus on a single disorder when asking people to participate. Instead, the *statistical analysis* of a particular disorder is performed, after those who have (or have had) it at baseline are excluded.

There are two types of cohort studies: **prospective** and **retrospective**. A prospective cohort study involves recruiting participants in the present

---

[#] 'unaffected' might be better, that is, they are unaffected by the disorder of interest.

A Concise Guide to Observational Studies in Healthcare, First Edition. Allan Hackshaw.
© 2015 John Wiley & Sons, Ltd. Published 2015 by John Wiley & Sons, Ltd.

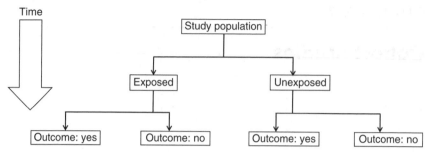

Figure 7.1 General design of a cohort study.

time, finding information about them now (or about their past), and then obtaining new data on them in the future.

A retrospective (or historical) cohort study sounds like a contradiction in terms, but it can be thought of as a prospective cohort that has already taken place. Participants are identified from existing records, including information about their characteristics, habits, and exposures, and then data on outcomes over a specified time period, perhaps up to the present day, are examined.

The obvious disadvantage of a retrospective cohort study is that only data that have already been collected can be used, so there is the potential for missing data, whereas in a prospective cohort study, the researchers can request the data they need and missing data can be minimised. A major advantage of a retrospective cohort study is that it can be performed much more quickly, because there is no requirement to wait several months or years to collect information on the outcome measures. Such studies are also often used to examine biological markers using stored samples (e.g. from biobanks associated with the study).

Prospective cohort studies are less easy to conduct than retrospective studies, because of the fundamental feature of regular contact with the study participants, either directly or indirectly, over several months or years. Many cohort studies, particularly those that are based on many participants from a relatively wide geographical location (e.g. nationally) do not have a single specific research objective. This is essentially to maximise the usefulness of the study, given the resources (staff and money) they require to set up and conduct. There may be research questions that only arise during the subsequent years, that were not apparent at the start of the study. Examples of well-known cohort studies are the British Doctors Study (established in 1951) [5] and the US Cancer Prevention Studies (I and II, which started in 1959 and 1982, respectively) [6]. All three have reported on a range of disorders over several decades, including different types of cancers, and cardiovascular disease.

Cohort studies could have a fixed accrual period, where participants are only asked to take part between certain dates (e.g. January–December 2005), or may be dynamic, in that people could take part any time. The fixed accrual period is most common, but dynamic accrual might be appropriate for studies based on, for example, hospital patients, in which it is easy to add to the cohort, and to follow them up.

Box 7.1 Examples of sampling frames and how participants were selected from them

Study objective	Sampling frame (eligibility)	How are participants selected
To examine the association between taking prenatal folic acid and the risk of having a child with autism spectrum disorder (ASD) [7]	All pregnant women in Norway who attended their routine ultrasound examination at about 18 weeks' gestation	All women were approached between 1999 and 2009
To examine how body weight changes over time in relation to diet and lifestyle activities [8]	The study was based on three established studies, each with their own sampling frame: (1) registered female nurses from 11 US states who were aged 30–55, (2) registered female nurses from 14 US states aged 25–42, and (3) registered male health professionals* aged 40–75 from 50 states. People who had obesity, diabetes, cancer, or cardiovascular, pulmonary, renal, or liver disease at baseline were excluded from the analysis	All were approached: (1) in 1976, (2) in 1989, and (3) in 1986
To examine the association between size of abdominal aorta and risk of death or hospital admission [9]	All men aged 65–74 who lived in Highland and Western Isles (Scotland) and attended the aortic aneurysm screening programme	All men who were screened between April 2001 and March 2004 were approached

* Dentists, pharmacists, optometrists, osteopath physicians, podiatrists, and veterinarians

As with all observational studies, a sampling frame must be used, and this should be representative of the target population of interest. Box 7.1 shows the sampling frames for three examples, covered in this chapter [7–9]. Boxes 7.2 to 7.4 illustrate key features of the examples, to highlight cohort studies in general.

When the exposed and unexposed participants are found within the same study population (i.e. sampling frame), this can be referred to as an **internal comparison**. However, it may be difficult to find a sufficient number of unexposed individuals in the cohort of interest. For example, if the research question is to examine the effect of coal dust on the risk of lung cancer among coal miners, all would be exposed. Therefore, an unexposed group must be found elsewhere, using a separate sampling frame, such as the general population, or perhaps another occupation. This can be referred to as an **external**

Box 7.2 Example of a cohort study where the outcome measure was based on counting people [7]

Objective: To examine whether taking folic acid supplements prenatally is associated with the risk of having a child with autism spectrum disorder (ASD).

Study participants: 85,176 children out of 97,179 and their mothers were eligible for the analysis (21,003 were excluded because there was no information on folic acid use, birthweight < 2500 g, multiple births, and gestational age < 32 weeks).

Location: National study conducted across Norway.

Design: The analysis on folic acid and ASD was part of an established prospective study (the Norwegian Mother and Child cohort, MoBa) examining a range of exposures and factors before and during pregnancy, and their influence on pregnancy outcomes. All pregnant women in Norway attending their 18 week ultrasound examination were asked to participate. Children were followed up for 7 years, with questionnaires sent to mothers when their baby was age 36 months and 5 and 7 years (from which cases of ASD were identified).

Exposure: Women who agreed to take part in the study completed questionnaires at 18 and 22 weeks' gestation. The survey at 18 weeks included questions about their intake of vitamins during the 4 weeks before the start of pregnancy and then in every 4-week block up to about 16 weeks. For the main analysis, 'exposed' was defined as any woman who took folic acid from 4 weeks before pregnancy up to 8 weeks after.

Outcome measure: Cases were detected via the questionaires and through hospital referrals and a national patient registry on all hospital and outpatient clinic diagnoses. ASD included (i) autistic disorder, (ii) Asperger syndrome, and (iii) pervasive developmental disorder not otherwise specified; all diagnosed using the *Diagnostic and Statistical Manual of Mental Disorders* (DSM, version IV). There were 270 cases of ASD in total.

Results: For the purpose of this analysis, follow-up data was up to March 2012. Table 7.1 shows the results.

Authors' conclusions: Prenatal folic acid use was associated with a lower risk of autistic disorder. Although the findings cannot establish causality, they do support prenatal folic acid supplementation.

---

comparison. It is important to avoid choosing an unexposed group that could lead to bias, which would under- or overestimate the association.

Once the sampling frame is identified, there may be no specific eligibility criteria. This was the case in the example on folic acid, in which all maternity units with >100 births annually were included, and all pregnant women who attended for the routine ultrasound examination were asked to take part. If eligibility criteria are to be applied, this may be done in two ways: at the start, when approaching participants, or for the analysis associated with a specific research objective. In the example of lifestyle habits (Box 7.3) and abdominal aorta size (Box 7.4), age at baseline was an inclusion criterion, so only people within a certain age range were invited to participate (Box 7.1). However, additional criteria were applied to the study of lifestyle habits when selecting

---

Box 7.3 Example of a cohort study where the outcome measure was based on 'taking measurements' on people [8]

Objective: To examine how body weight changes over time in relation to diet and lifestyle activities such as exercise.

Study participants: 120,877 men and women aged ≤65, who were participating in one of three national prospective cohort studies. Participants who had chronic diseases (including cancer, diabetes, and cardiovascular, pulmonary, renal, or liver disease) or were obese were excluded from the statistical analysis. Also, they had to have complete data on body weight and lifestyle factors at baseline.

Location: Female registered nurses from 11 US states (Nurses' Health Study (NHS) and from 14 states (Nurses' Health Study II (NHS II)), and registered male health professionals from all 50 US states (Health Professionals Follow-up Study (HPFS)).

Design: The three studies are established longitudinal cohorts examining a range of exposure and outcomes, focussing on cancer and cardiovascular disease. Details of diet and lifestyle characteristics were obtained through self-completed questionnaires sent to participants every 2 years. The follow-up period was 20 years for the NHS and HPFS and 12 years for NHS II.

Exposure: For the purposes of this statistical analysis, data were used from questionnaires completed every 4 years. Several exposures were examined in the article. Diet was measured as servings per day of specific food and drink items. Other lifestyle characteristics used as exposures were smoking, exercise, sleep, and time spent watching television, each based on usage or time spent per day.

Outcome measure: Body weight (in pounds) was self-reported and recorded on the regular questionnaires, corresponding with the diet and lifestyle questionnaires (i.e. every 4 years for this analysis). The main outcome was the change in body weight over a 4-year period; and this was pooled (averaged) across several 4-year periods during the observed length of follow-up.

Results: See Table 7.2 and Figure 7.4.

Authors' conclusions: Some dietary factors, physical activity, smoking, amount of sleep, and time spent watching TV are each independently associated with long-term weight gain, and there is a substantial aggregate effect.

---

the data for the *analyses* (i.e. after follow-up), in which people who had certain existing disorders at baseline were excluded (Box 7.3).

If investigating causality, a key strength of cohort studies is ensuring that an exposure came *before* the disorder of interest (Box 2.6). There is no reason to recruit or analyse people who already had the disorder at baseline. In the three examples in this chapter, the outcome measures were children with ASD (Box 7.2), change in body weight (Box 7.3), or death/hospital admission (Box 7.4). In the first and third examples, it is clear that the exposures came (and were measured) before the outcomes. In the second example, the change in body weight was recorded at the same time as changes in diet, when each could be compared with the baseline values.

Box 7.4 Example of a cohort study where the outcome measure was based on time-to-event data [9]

Objective: To examine the association between the size of the abdominal aorta and hospital admission and mortality.

Study participants: Men aged 65–74 who attended screening for aortic aneurysm. 8355 men attended screening (representing 90% of those who were invited), and of these, 8146 completed a baseline questionnaire, allowing their records to be linked to a morbidity and mortality registry for follow-up data.

Location: Men residing in the Highland and Western Isles, Scotland, who were screened between 2001 and 2004.

Design: A self-completed questionnaire collected data on characteristics such as place of birth, deprivation, smoking status, personal and family history of cardiovascular disease, and general health.

Exposure: Size of the abdominal aorta.

Outcome measures: Cause of death and first admission to hospital (and the reason for this). These data were obtained using the Scottish Morbidity Record Database. Cause of death was classified according to the International Classification of Diseases (ICD), 9th and 10th revisions. Follow-up was to June 2010.

Results: Table 7.3 shows selected baseline characteristics, and selected results are given in Table 7.4 and Figure 7.5.

Authors' conclusions: Men with a large abdominal aorta are more likely to be admitted to hospital for cardiovascular disease and die early.

7.3 Measuring variables, exposures, and outcome measures

In a cohort study, exposures and other factors are measured at baseline, and outcome measures are ascertained over the subsequent months or years. The most common type of cohort study analysis is of the association between the baseline information and the outcomes. However, some exposures, for example, diet and lifestyle (Box 7.3), could change over time, especially if there is a long follow-up period. If this is likely to occur, the exposures should be measured during follow-up (called **longitudinal cohort study**). Interest would be in how *changes* in diet and lifestyle over time influence the outcome measures (such as cardiovascular disease). Figure 10.1 is an example in which using only baseline exposure information could lead to a diluted effect if the exposure status significantly changes during a long follow-up period. Principles covered in Section 5.3 also apply to cohort studies.

Cohort studies are commonly used to estimate risk, that is, the chance of having a defined event (e.g. stopped smoking), of developing a specific disorder, or of death. Studies of risk such as these could use two types of outcome measures: 'counting people' and time-to-event data. However, there are also cohort studies that aim to examine how certain outcomes change over time (e.g. measures of blood pressure or body weight), and for these, there is no concept of risk.[#]

[#] Unless the measurement is categorised, in which case interest is then in, for example, the risk of having high blood pressure (that exceeds a pre-defined cut-off).

Exposures and outcome measures should be measured using the same methods for all participants, and when determining the outcome measure, it is best to use standard and validated criteria where possible. An established method for cause of death is the World Health Organisation ICD. Non-standard methods developed specifically for a study require careful explanation and justification, and if the method has been developed and then tested on the same dataset, there is a possibility of bias. Independent assessment of the outcome measure for all individuals may strengthen the reliability of the findings, that is, assessment by someone who does not know the exposure status of the participant or is not directly involved in the research study team (but this can be expensive to do).

7.4 Collecting the data

Data for cohort studies can be collected in a similar way to case–control studies (Section 6.4) or cross-sectional studies (Section 5.4). Unlike some case–control and cross-sectional studies, in which a proxy could provide data for the study instead of the participant, it is usual for cohort studies to obtain information directly from the participants (particularly the baseline information). The three examples in this chapter show that data were collected in a variety of ways (Figure 7.2). Prospective cohort studies require significant resources, so efficient methods are needed to capture data, especially during follow-up

Exposure:	Folic acid	Diet and lifestyle	Abdominal aorta size
Outcome measure:	Autism spectrum disorder (ASD)	Body weight	Mortality and hospital admission
Type of outcome:	'Counting people'	'Taking measurements on people'	Time-to-event
Baseline (exposure):	Self-completed questionnaire	Self-completed questionnaire	• Ultrasound scan • Self-completed questionnaire
During follow up:		Self-completed questionnaire every 4 years	
End of study (outcomes):	3–10 years later* • Self-completed questionnaire • National registry data • Confirmation of ASD diagnosis by central research team	12 or 20 years later* Self-reported body weight, every 4 years	6–9 years later* National registry data

* Approximately after baseline.

Figure 7.2 How data were collected in the three cohort studies used as examples in this chapter. 'National registry data' do not directly involve the study participant.

which can last for several years. Attempting to collect data regularly requires a balance of objectives:

- Frequent collection would be expensive, and participants may become less interested, though this approach would be less affected by having to recall information from memory.
- Infrequent collection is cheaper, but there is a loss of information in how the exposures and/or outcome measures change over time, and people may forget exposures/outcomes since the last assessment.

Self-completed questionnaires during follow-up are an efficient way of requesting large amounts of information but non-responders and incomplete responders are likely. Telephone surveys, where the researcher works through the questionnaire items with the study participant, could overcome this, but these require staff (increasing costs) and often a shorter questionnaire, because participants are unlikely to want to spend much more than an hour going through a survey by telephone.

In the future, cohort studies are likely to involve more information technology (see page 19).

There are two major problems with prospective cohort studies, which often increase with longer follow-up and can have an impact on the study size available for the statistical analyses and therefore reliability of the results:

1. **People who are lost to follow-up**: They often move address or do not respond to correspondence, and the researchers cannot trace them. This problem is difficult to overcome, particularly if people move abroad. Participants could be reminded during follow-up to inform the research team if they move.
2. **People who withdraw**, that is, those who decide to not continue in the study: All participants have a right to withdraw at any time; however, reasons for this could be ascertained. It could be lack of interest, lack of perceived personal benefit, or the assessments have become burdensome. If the latter arises, it is important to still be allowed access to medical records (and registry data) if used to provide outcome data, because individuals often agree to this.

These two features are different. Obtaining outcome measures on those lost to follow-up is usually impossible, but this is not necessarily the case for those who withdraw.

7.5 Sample size

The three examples used in this chapter are each based on many study participants. Although it is possible to conduct relatively smaller studies, for example, from a single centre in which there may only be 100 individuals to follow up, the size and duration of follow-up must still be sufficient to address the study objectives.

Many cohort studies are already ongoing, with fixed numbers of participants and events, so a sample size calculation for a specific research objective might have limited value or not done, as in two examples covered in this chapter [8,9]. However, if a sample size were estimated, and the target number of participants and/or events far exceeded that observed in the study, the researchers may still wish to proceed with the analysis.

Information needed for sample size estimation when examining associations

The principles of sample size estimation for cohort studies are similar to those for case–control studies (see Section 6.5). When the outcome measure is based on 'counting people' or time-to-event data, the number of events is important, often more so than the total number of participants in the study. Therefore, although it might be easy to conduct a small cohort study, finding no or few events would not provide useful information (wide 95% confidence intervals and large p-values). If the number of participants recruited is limited, extending the follow-up may increase the number of events. There is, therefore, a relationship between target sample size, expected event rate, length of follow-up, and available resources that need to be considered by researchers.

When there is a single exposure factor of interest and a single outcome measure (e.g. disorder), several pieces of information are needed for the sample size calculation (Figure 7.3). Items such as the percentage of participants who are expected to be exposed and the percentage of the unexposed group who would have the outcome should ideally come from prior information but other times are simply best guesses. Statistical packages have sample size facilities, and there are software programmes [10, 11], including those freely available for observational studies [12].

For example, in the folic acid study, Box 7.2, the study size of 85,176 had 93, 73 and 45% power to detect odds ratios of 0.50, 0.60 and 0.70 respectively, assuming 68% of the participants were exposed (ie. mothers took folic acid) and ASD prevalence of 0.13%.

Drop outs could be allowed for in the sample size. For example, if the calculation produced a study size of 1000 participants and 15% are expected to be lost during follow-up (there is no measure of the endpoint on them), the target size could be inflated to 1180 [85% of 1180 is 1000, where $1180 = 1000/(1 - 0.15)$].

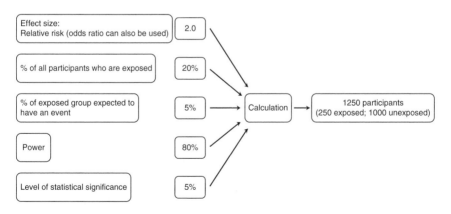

Sample size increases with any of the following:
effect size gets closer to the no effect value; % exposed decreases; % with event decreases.

Figure 7.3 Information required for a sample size estimation for cohort studies in which the effect size is a relative risk.

7.6 Analysing data and interpreting results

When the outcome measure is based on 'counting people' or time-to-events, the concept of risk is used. Unlike cross-sectional or case–control studies, cohort studies can be used to estimate the incidence of a disorder. When considering the influence of potential confounding factors, the same approaches are used as covered in Chapter 6 (including Figure 6.3).

7.7 Outcome measures based on 'counting people' endpoints: Folic acid and ASD (Box 7.2)

Measuring variables, exposures, and outcome measures

In most studies, the participant is obvious and is almost always a single individual. However, in this example, the 'participant' was a mother/child pair. The mother was recruited and provided exposure information, but the outcome measure was obtained on the child, during follow-up. It is possible that a woman could have had more than one pregnancy during the recruitment period of 2002–2008 and so be counted more than once.

The original study aimed to examine several factors associated with the mothers and outcome of pregnancy (the child and mother), so there was no single research objective. But the exposure of interest in this particular analysis was folic acid supplementation. Women were recruited to the study at 18 weeks of pregnancy, but the survey given at the time requested details about folic acid intake as far back as 4 weeks before the start of pregnancy, requiring them to remember their intake over the past 5–6 months, including intake in each 4-week interval up to 18 weeks. It is possible that many women were still continuing supplementation to 18 weeks, making it easier to recall this information accurately. To simplify matters, women were only asked whether or not they took folic acid, rather than the amount taken. Recall bias (Box 1.6) would not occur in this situation, because women had not yet given birth, so there should not be a differential report in folic acid use between those with children with ASD and those who were unaffected.

The outcome measure of interest was the diagnosis of ASD, of which there were three types: autistic disorder, Asperger syndrome, and 'pervasive developmental disorder not otherwise specified'. Children suspected to have ASD were initially identified using the questionnaires sent to mothers during follow-up, or from a national hospital registry (to which the study participants could be linked), which indicated that the child had already been diagnosed with ASD. The child was then invited for a clinical assessment, and ASD was diagnosed or confirmed using standard and validated criteria, based on the evaluation as well as information from parents and teachers. This approach attempted to maximise the number of affected individuals assessed in the same way, and it used an independent assessment of ASD diagnosis. Importantly, the clinical assessment was conducted without knowledge of the exposure status of the mother/child.

Analysing data and interpreting results

The outcome measure (chance of having a child with ASD) was analysed using a **logistic regression** (see page 69).

What are the main results?
Published results should usually include a table showing the study participants by baseline characteristics <u>and</u> according to exposure status (if appropriate).[#] There are two reasons for this:
1. To describe the group of individuals in the study, because the conclusions will often be influenced by how representative they are of the target
   population of interest.
2. To show whether or not the exposed and unexposed groups have very
   different characteristics (these two groups should be 'the same' in order
   to make reliable conclusions about risk and causal factors; see Chapter 1,
   page 5). If there are big differences for some factors, these need to be
   allowed (adjusted) for in the statistical analysis as potential confounding
   factors.
In this study, there were clear baseline differences between the exposed and
unexposed groups:
• Maternal education: 13.6% (no folic acid) versus 4.9% (folic acid) had < 12
  years of education; and 15.0 versus 26.7% had ≥17 years.
• Number of previous pregnancies: 38.4% (no folic acid) versus 47.0% (folic
  acid) who had no prior pregnancies; and 26.4 versus 16.6% for those who
  had ≥2 prior pregnancies.

The main results are shown in Table 7.1. The investigators analysed each
type of ASD separately; it is always useful to show both the number of study
participants and number of events in each exposure group. The effect size
for this type of outcome measure is the odds ratio (OR). Although researchers can calculate relative risks from cohort studies, this study was analysed
using logistic regression because confounding factors can be adjusted for.
Logistic regression analysis works with OR, which can usually be interpreted in a similar way to relative risks, unless the disorder is common (see
Table 3.2).
   In this study, the unadjusted OR was 0.51 (49% risk reduction), indicating a
halving of the risk of having a child with autistic disorder among women who
took folic acid, compared with those who did not. This is a large effect. The
adjusted OR becomes 0.61 (39% risk reduction), and still represents a clinically
important effect. The potential confounding factors had only relatively small
effect on the association between folic acid use and risk of autistic disorder.
Reporting both the unadjusted and adjusted effect sizes is useful, in order to
demonstrate the influence of potential confounders. The results for Asperger
syndrome suggested a decreased risk by 35% (OR 0.65).
   Table 7.1 also shows the OR according to when women started to take folic
acid (i.e. whether the ORs decreased or increased). It is plausible that women
who took folic acid for the longest would have had the greatest reduction in
risk, but there was no such obvious trend here. However, a major problem
with this analysis is that each subgroup was based on relatively few events, so
there was no clear pattern.

[#] An example is shown in Table 7.3.

Table 7.1 OR between two types of autistic spectrum disorder and folic acid use.

	Number of ASD cases (total number of children)	OR (95% CI)
Autistic disorder		
No folic acid used	50 (24,134)	1.0 (reference group)
Folic acid used	64 (61,042)	0.51 (0.35–0.73), unadjusted
		0.61 (0.41–0.90), adjusted*
Started folic acid		
4–1 week before pregnant	32 (28,061)	0.67 (0.40–1.14), adjusted*
1–4 weeks after pregnant	18 (16,797)	0.58 (0.32–1.05)*
5–8 weeks after	14 (16,184)	0.44 (0.23–0.83)*
9–16 weeks after	18 (9395)	0.87 (0.49–1.57)*
Asperger syndrome		
No folic acid used	27 (12,899)	1.0 (reference group)
Folic acid used	21 (17,218)	0.65 (0.36–1.16), adjusted

*For year of birth, maternal education, and the number of previous pregnancies.

What could the true effect be, given that the study was conducted on a sample of people?

The 95% CI for autistic disorder was 0.41–0.90 (Table 7.1). The true OR is likely to be somewhere between 0.41 (59% reduction) and 0.90 (10% reduction), and the best estimate was 0.61 (39% risk reduction). The CI is quite wide, considering the large study size; however, the width is determined by the standard error, which is influenced by both study size and number of events (Box 3.8). In this example, there were 85,176 participants (mother/child pairs), but the number of autistic disorder cases (events), 114, was relatively small. Nevertheless, the results are sufficiently reliable to make a conclusion. For Asperger syndrome, the 95% CI was also quite wide (0.36–1.16), but this is again unsurprising, given the relatively low number of cases (48). The interval includes the no effect value, so there is a possibility that the true OR for this group was 1.0.

Could the observed result be a chance finding in this particular study?

No p-values were reported in the published paper, but because the 95% CI excludes the no effect value (OR of 1.0), the p-value must be <0.05 (Figure 3.7). The observed OR of 0.61 is unlikely to be due to chance and is probably a real effect. In addition, the upper limit (0.90) is relatively far from the no effect value, so the p-value is likely to be fairly small. Using Box 6.8 the estimated p-value is 0.01.

How good is the evidence?

The adjusted OR indicated a moderate/large effect, and design strengths of the study included the large number of participants, prospective collection of outcome measures, and a combination of methods to ascertain ASD. The authors considered some limitations:

- There might have been confounders (unknown or not measured) that were not allowed for, which could explain the association of folic acid

supplementation with autistic disorder. However, there was another expo-sure (prenatal fish oil supplements), which had similar associations with maternal characteristics as with folic acid. If there were other factors that explain the association, similar OR should have been seen for fish oil, but the OR was 1.29 for users versus non-users.
• The number of ASD cases was lower than expected, indicating possible under-ascertainment. The problem was not considered to be important for autistic disorder, because case ascertainment was close to complete for older children (born 2002–2004), and among these, the OR for the associa-tion was still strong (0.45).
There was independent evidence from a case–control study that found a lower risk of ASD among women who took prenatal folic acid, and there was already established biological evidence of the beneficial effect of this vitamin on neural tube development including a randomized clinical trial of folic acid and pre-vention [13]. Although the authors of the cohort study found an association, they could not establish causality, which is an appropriate conclusion to make.

7.8 Outcome measures based on 'taking measurements on people' endpoints: Lifestyle habits and body weight (Box 7.3)

Measuring variables, exposures, and outcome measures

In this example, the main outcome measure was body weight, which represents continuous data, so there is no direct concept of risk. The purpose was to see how these measures changed, over time, as the exposures changed. This is a type of cohort study called a **longitudinal study**. If the researchers had wanted to examine risk, they would have had to categorise weight, for example, <100 and ≥100 kg, and the analysis would then have been based on the proportion (risk) of participants who weighed ≥100 kg. Although this approach is easy, information on the variability in body weight is lost in the statistical analysis.

There were many exposures, based on specific dietary items and lifestyle habits including daily intake of fruits, vegetables, and alcohol, as well as phys-ical activity, and amount of sleep. Some of these were relatively easy to quan-tify (e.g. number of hours of sleep per day). However, measuring the dietary items was complex as they are a mixture of solids and liquids, and the amount consumed for each type varied considerably. Using the weight of each item as a measure is impractical, requiring the study participants to weigh (or guess the weight of) the amount of food they consume. The unit of measure chosen for the study was 'servings per day'. This might appear imprecise, but it indi-cated what a typical person might consume, in accepted units. For example, a serving of potato chips could be a bag, and a serving of fruit could be an orange. The questionnaires were detailed, but an advantage of using health professionals as study participants is that they would be familiar with the topic, and so may complete the questionnaires more reliably than people from the general population.

Body weight was also self-reported by the participants, and measured sev-eral times during follow-up (Figure 7.2). A bias could arise if those with the highest weights were more likely to under-report their weight or report a more favourable diet, which could underestimate the association between diet and weight. To determine whether this bias was present, the body weight of a sample of study participants was measured by researchers, and found to be highly correlated with the self-reported weights.

Analysing data and interpreting results
In this study the outcome measure, body weight, can be analysed using **linear regression** (Chapter 3, page 66).

What are the main results?
Unlike the other two examples in this chapter, in which the exposure was a single, categorical factor, in this study, there were many exposures, so it was not possible to report the baseline characteristics according to exposed and unexposed groups. Instead, the baseline characteristics table in the published paper provides a summary of the key dietary and lifestyle factors in each of the groups used in the paper.

Table 7.2 shows the main results for selected exposures (dietary items). Each item is included in the regression as a continuous measure, without being put into categories, and so a linear relationship is assumed between the dietary item and change in body weight. The effect size for each factor (obtained from the linear regression) was the change in body weight over a 4-year period. As expected, there were many potential confounding factors, and each effect size for a dietary item was adjusted for all other items. Allowing for so many factors is usually only reliable for large datasets; in smaller datasets, the regression model could 'break down', which could be indicated by very large or small effect sizes or CI limits (may appear as infinity). The results in this study can be assessed by examining whether the effect size materially changes after adjustment, and whether it moves closer or further away from the no effect value (Figure 6.3).

Table 7.2 Change in body weight (in pounds) over a 4-year period (averaged across several 4-year periods) in relation to selected dietary items.

Increased consumption of 1 serving per day	Weight change (pounds) (95% CI), p-value	
	Allowing for age only	Allowing for many factors*
Fruits	−0.69 (−0.92, −0.46) p<0.001	−0.49 (−0.63, −0.35) p<0.001
Nuts	−0.78 (−1.31, −0.26) p<0.001	−0.57 (−0.97, −0.17) p=0.005
Potato chips	+3.01 (2.09, 3.94) p<0.001	+1.69 (1.30, 2.09) p<0.001
French fries	+6.59 (4.35, 8.83) p<0.001	+3.35 (2.29, 4.42) p<0.001
Low-fat dairy foods	−0.17 (−0.21, −0.13) p<0.001	−0.05 (−0.14, 0.05) p=0.33
Cheese	0.13 (−0.08, 0.34) p=0.23	0.02 (−0.09, 0.13) p=0.75

To convert pounds to kilograms, multiply the results by 0.45.
A negative sign indicates weight loss from baseline; a positive sign is weight gain.
*Age, baseline body mass index, sleep duration, and changes (from baseline) in physical activity, alcohol consumption, television watching, smoking, and all other dietary items.

The results in Table 7.2 can be interpreted as follows:
- For every extra serving of fruit consumed each day, body weight reduced by 0.69 pounds over a 4-year period after allowing for age only. The effect after allowing for all other factors was a weight reduction of 0.49 pounds (0.22 kg), indicating that some, but not all, of the effect of the 0.69 pound loss was due to other (confounding) factors.
- The largest weight reduction was associated with increasing the intake of nuts by 1 serving per day: –0.57 pounds (–0.26 kg).
- The largest weight increase was seen for french fries. Each extra serving, per day, led to a weight increase of 6.59 pounds (3.0 kg) over 4 years, but about half of this effect was due to confounding factors; the adjusted effect size was 3.35 pounds (1.5 kg). There was a similar finding for potato chips (i.e. the effect was approximately halved, from 3.01 to 1.69 pounds.).
- A small/moderate weight loss was seen for consumption of low-fat dairy foods (–0.17 pounds), but this became almost no effect after allowing for other factors (–0.05).
- There was little/no association for cheese, either before or after adjustment.

These changes in weight might appear relatively small, in the context of gains or losses over a 4-year period, but they were associated with only one extra serving, per day, of one food item. Additional servings of the same food item, and the effects of other food/drink items, are therefore likely to have a cumulative effect on weight. It was unexpected that eating more fruit or nuts could lead to weight loss, because both add calories. It is possible that people who ate fruit and nuts reduced their intake of other foods with high calorific content, thus decreasing their total energy intake, which led to the small/moderate weight loss.

Figure 7.4 shows the independent effects of diet and physical activity on changes in body weight. Diet was quantified as an overall score, based on changes in each food/drink item. As expected, people with the 'worst' diet and the least amount of physical activity had the largest weight gain, on average almost 6 pounds over 4 years, compared with those in the highest category. The figure shows that food consumption and exercise had independent effects. By holding one category of diet constant (so that people had similar diet scores, and therefore diet would not act as a confounder), weight increased with decreasing physical activity (i.e. as the quintile moved from 5 to 1). The same pattern was seen when holding a category of physical activity constant.

What could the true effect be, given that the study was conducted on a sample of people?
Table 7.2 shows the 95% CIs for each food item. The width for some of these intervals, such as the adjusted weight change for fruits and low-fat dairy foods, was narrow, partly due to the large study size. The food item that had the largest effect on body weight was french fries, and the results indicate that the *true* weight change could have been as low as 2.29 pounds (1 kg) or as much as 4.42 pounds (2.0 kg), although it is more likely to lie around the middle of the interval. As with the point estimates of the effect sizes given earlier, the important consideration is whether the *adjusted* 95% confidence limits

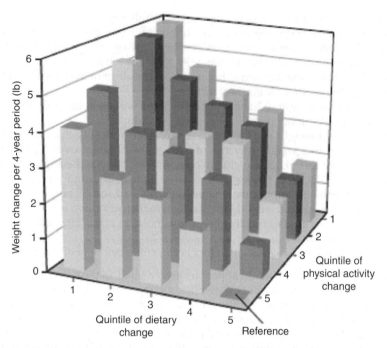

Figure 7.4 How body weight changes in relation to changes in diet and physical activity. Each food/drink item had a score , and a total score for 'diet' was calculated for each participant. A low quintile for diet indicates the 20% of participants who tend to have the 'worst' diets (i.e. consume foods or drinks that increase weight), and a low quintile for physical activity indicates the 20% of people who perform the least amount of physical activity. Source: Mozaffarian et al. 2011 [8]. Reproduced by permission of Massachusetts Medical Society.

approach or overlap the no effect value (Figure 6.3), because this would provide evidence that the factor was not independently associated with change in body weight. In Table 7.2, this was observed for low-fat dairy foods, where the unadjusted upper limit was −0.13 but became +0.05 after adjustment, so there was the possibility that the true effect was no weight change (zero).

Could the observed result be a chance finding in this particular study?
The p-values for the adjusted effect sizes were small for fruits, nuts, potato chips, and french fries (all $p < 0.001$). This indicates that the observed changes in weight were each highly unlikely to be due to chance. Small p-values such as these often tend to be associated with large effects, but in this example (where the effects are relatively small/moderate) are due to the very large sample size. The p-values for cheese support the conclusion that this has little/no effect on body weight. However, we can see that the p-value for low-fat dairy foods changed from <0.001 unadjusted (strong evidence for an effect) to 0.33 adjusted (little/no evidence), confirming the importance of allowing for potential confounders when making conclusions about risk factors (exposures).

How good is the evidence?
The obvious strength of this study was the large sample size. Many food and drink items were examined, and the effect sizes for several remained high or low, and statistically significant, after allowing for all other dietary items and lifestyle factors. Another strength was that the investigators showed the results were generally consistent, and quantitatively similar, across the three cohorts (different groups of individuals, and men or women), important for considering causality (see Box 2.6). As with any very large study or when many factors are examined, it is possible to find results that are unexpected, or without biological plausibility, even when they are statistically significant (e.g. the weight loss associated with increasing intake of fruits, nuts, and yogurt). While some findings might lead to further investigations elsewhere, some could still be due to chance[#].

Potential limitations in this study were as follows: (i) accuracy of measuring food and drink items by self-report, and (ii) given the complexity of a combination of diet, lifestyle, and other habits that can contribute to body weight, there may have been additional confounding factors that were not measured and for which allowance could not be made. Because the study participants were health professionals, the findings might not be applicable to a general population. However, although the actual amounts of certain foods and drinks are likely to differ between the participants and people in general, it is possible that the *change* in body weight (the effect size) for a given *change* in diet would be similar.

The findings were generally consistent with what was expected and with independent evidence from other studies. The authors conclude that targeting diet and lifestyle factors could help prevent obesity, confirming what was known already.

7.9 Outcome measures based on time-to-event endpoints: Abdominal aorta size and hospital admission and mortality (Box 7.4)

Measuring variables, exposures, and outcome measures
This cohort study had a focussed objective, to link the result of a single screening test with specific health outcomes. Two separate sources of data were used. The participants self-completed a baseline questionnaire when they attended for screening, providing details about their personal and family history, following which there was no further direct contact with them. The outcome measures were obtained using national databases, from which the study participants who had given consent could be linked (Figure 7.2).

The exposure was the maximum size of the abdominal aorta (anteroposterior diameter), measured using an ultrasound scan. This is a standard measurement and can be considered objective.

[#] A p-value of 0.001 still means that there is a very small possibility (1 in 1000 similar studies) that the observed result could be a chance finding, that is, there really is no effect.

The outcome measures were cause of death and reasons for the first hospital admission following the screening test.

Analysing data and interpreting results

The outcome measure in this study, time to death or time to first hospital admission (after screening), can be analysed using **Cox regression** (page 69).

What are the main results?

In a randomised clinical trial, a table of baseline characteristics shows whether the randomisation process produced similar exposed (new intervention) and unexposed (control) groups. Major differences are unexpected. However, such differences can occur in observational studies (because there has been no randomisation), and the factors may need to be allowed for in the statistical analysis as potential confounders.

Table 7.3 shows selected baseline characteristics for the example. The exposure variable (size of abdominal aorta) was a continuous measurement that was categorised using standard cut-offs, allowing the data to be easily displayed, though this meant that the groups were of unequal size. The definition of such categories should always be specified. If there are no generally accepted groupings, objective approaches should be used (see Box 7.5).

In each group, the factors must sum to 100%; so for males with aortic diameters 25–29 mm the sum of the percentage who were never-smokers, former smokers, or current smokers was $21.7 + 53.2 + 25.1 = 100$. Assessing baseline differences can be made by comparing the percentages, means or medians of the factors, and judging any differences appear large, with supporting evidence from p-values (last column of Table 7.3). Using p-values alone could flag differences that are not clinically meaningful, and a small p-value might

Table 7.3 Selected baseline characteristics in each exposure group (size of abdominal aorta) from the study in Box 7.4.

	Size of abdominal aorta at screening			p-value*
	≤24 mm N = 7063	25–29 mm N = 669	≥30 mm N = 414	
Mean age (years)	70.3	70.6	70.8	<0.001
Smoking status (%)				<0.001
Never	32.3	21.7	14.3	
Former	50.4	53.2	54.1	
Current	17.2	25.1	31.6	
Close relative ever had stroke (%)				0.20
Yes	19.5	19.7	16.2	
No	73.7	74.1	75.8	
Missing data	6.8	6.1	8.0	

* p-value for the association between the factor and size of abdominal aorta.

Box 7.5 Categorising continuous measurements in a cohort study

Common groupings are based on the median, tertiles, quartiles, or quintiles (see page 76), and each of these can produce one of the following:
1. Similar number of study participants in each group
2. Similar number of events in each group
3. Similar number of unexposed participants in each group
4. Similar number of exposed participants in each group
An advantage of (2) is that each group contains a sufficient number of events, to improve the precision (standard errors) of the effect sizes.

An advantage of (3) and (4) is that the categorisation is based on a homogenous group of participants in terms of exposure status. They should produce a clearer association between the exposure and outcome measure.

---

only really be due to having a (very) large study. This initially appears to be the case with age, where the p-value is <0.001, but the difference between the lowest and highest mean age is only 0.5 years (70.8–70.3). The question is whether a 6-month difference in age at baseline could really be associated with a noticeable increase in the abdominal aorta and also the outcomes. There was a clear association with smoking status, with more current smokers in the highest size group compared with the lowest group (31.6 vs. 17.2%). Because it is also known that smokers are more likely to die or be admitted to hospital, this was an obvious confounding factor. There was little evidence of an association between the exposure status and family history of stroke.

The risk of hospital admission for circulatory disease, according to the exposure group, is shown graphically in Figure 7.5. There is a clear trend in the curves and none of them cross or overlap. Although these curves are based on data unadjusted for confounders, they are always worth providing. Without the curves, it is not possible to see how risk changes over time, or between groups.

Table 7.4 shows the unadjusted and adjusted hazard ratios. Allowance was made for the deprivation score, even though it was not statistically significantly associated with the exposure. Allowance should be made for a combination of factors that are already known to be confounders (whether or not the p-values for these factors are small in the study being analysed), and those where there seems to be an association in the particular study. If the study is large enough (and has a sufficient number of events), it is often better to adjust for too many, rather than too few, factors to avoid doubt over whether the adjustment has been adequate:
- The unadjusted risk of dying from any cause was higher in both the 25–29 and ≥30 mm groups (1.46, 46% increase in risk, and 2.57, 157% increase in risk), but both decreased after adjustment for the potential confounders, especially among men with aortas 25–29 mm, indicating little association in this group (1.08). The adjusted hazard ratio for men with aortas ≥30 mm was still high (2.03, i.e. a doubling of the risk of dying).
- The risk of hospital admission for circulatory disease was clinically significant for both aorta size groups and after adjustment for confounding.

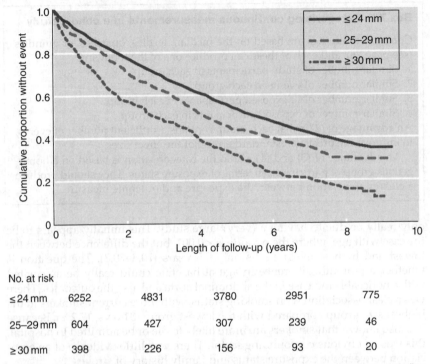

No. at risk

≤24 mm	6252	4831	3780	2951	775
25–29 mm	604	427	307	239	46
≥30 mm	398	226	156	93	20

Figure 7.5 Kaplan–Meier curves for time to hospital admission for circulatory disease, according to size of the abdominal aorta. Source: Duncan et al. 2012 [9]. Reproduced by permission of BMJ Publishing Ltd.

Table 7.4 Hazard ratios for cause of death and first admission to hospital according to abdominal aorta size group (number of events shown in brackets).

	Reference group	Unadjusted hazard ratio (95% CI)		Adjusted hazard ratio (95% CI)*	
	≤24 mm N=7063	25–29 mm N=669	≥30 mm N=414	25–29 mm N=669	≥30 mm N=414
All-cause mortality	1.0 (512)	1.46 (1.05–2.02) (69)	2.57 (1.86–3.55) (73)	1.08 (0.73–1.59)	2.03 (1.40–2.94)
Hospital admission for circulatory disease	1.0 (3796)	1.24 (1.09–1.42) (406)	1.92 (1.65–2.22) (329)	1.20 (1.04–1.39)	1.51 (1.27–1.79)

for age; number of pack-years smoked; deprivation score; general health score; personal history of heart attack, high blood pressure, or stroke; and close relative with history of aortic aneurysm.

In the published paper, several other outcomes were discussed (including cancer and hospital admission for diabetes). However, care should be taken when attempting to interpret too many endpoints, especially if the corresponding number of events is small.

What could the true effect be, given that the study was conducted on a sample of people?
As with the point estimates given earlier, the important consideration is whether the 95% CIs approach or overlap the no effect value, after adjustment for the confounding factors. For hospital admission, all 95% CIs for both aorta size groups excluded the no effect value, even after adjustment for confounders. For all-cause mortality, only the ≥30 mm group had a 95% CI like this, with a lower limit that is still clinically meaningful (hazard ratio 1.40, 40% increase in deaths).

Could the observed result be a chance finding in this particular study?
No p-values were reported in this article, but some are expected to be small (<0.01), because they have large effects sizes, and the 95% CIs are far from the no effect value (see Figure 3.7). But both outcomes in Table 7.4 among men with an aorta ≥30 mm had 95% CIs that excluded 1.0, reflecting a real effect. Using Box 6.8, an estimate of the p-values (which should be reasonably close to those from the Cox regression analysis) are 0.002 (mortality, hazard ratio 2.03) and $p < 0.0001$ (hospital admission, hazard ratio 1.51).

How good is the evidence?
The study was reasonably large (8146 men), of whom the number with an event was also sufficiently large to produce reliable results for the main analyses (654 deaths and 4531 hospital admissions for circulatory disease). Other strengths included a homogenous population of men (same geographical region), high uptake of screening (the 8146 men represented 86% of all men living in that region at the time), and allowance for many potential confounders (involving factors associated with the men or disease history of close relatives).

There were only 11 deaths due to an aneurysm (0.14% after 10 years), low compared with two other studies (0.33 and 0.41%). The authors could not explain this, except to postulate that the difference might be due to better cardiovascular risk prevention in these men. However, the association between risk of cardiovascular disease and aorta size is consistent with what was known already.

Men with aortas ≥30 mm should already be part of a routine follow-up plan, so the results of this article confirmed the importance of this. In addition, the authors recommended that men with aortas 25–29 mm should have health education to control their risk factors or additional screening.

7.10 Key points

• Cohort studies are generally the preferred approach to evaluating the effect of an exposure (risk factor) on an outcome, especially for assessing causality.

- Eligibility criteria can be applied at the start (i.e. who is invited to participate) or at the end (i.e. who is included in a particular statistical analysis).
- All participants should be assessed and managed in the same way during follow-up, to avoid bias.
- Loss to follow-up and withdrawals can lead to missing data, especially for the main outcome measures, and should be allowed for in the sample size calculation.
- Data can come directly from participants or medical records or by flagging them with regional or national databases/registries.
- When examining risk factors and causality, important potential confounders should be allowed for in the statistical analysis.
- The interpretation of effect sizes such as relative risk, OR, mean difference, and hazard ratio (and 95% CIs and p-values) is the same as in other chapters.

References

1. Silman AJ, Macfarlane GJ. *Epidemiological Studies: A Practical Guide.* Cambridge University Press. Second Edition (2002).
2. Rothman KJ. *Epidemiology: An Introduction.* Oxford University Press. First Edition (2002).
3. dos Santos Silva I. Cohort studies. In: *Cancer Epidemiology: Principles and Methods.* IARC Press (1999). http://www.iarc.fr/en/publications/pdfs-online/epi/cancerepi/. Accessed 19 May 2014.
4. Schulz KF, Grimes DA. Cohort studies: marching towards outcomes. *Lancet* 2002;359:341–5.
5. Doll R, Peto R, Boreham J, Sutherland I. Mortality in relation to smoking: 50 years' observation on male British doctors. *BMJ* 2004;328(7455):1519. doi:10.1136/bmj.38142.554479.AE
6. US Cancer Prevention Studies (I and II). http://www.cancer.org/research/researchto-preventcancer/index. Accessed 19 May 2014.
7. Surén P, Roth C, Bresnahan M, Haugen M, Hornig M, Hirtz D, et al. Association between maternal use of folic acid supplements and risk of autism spectrum disorders in children. *JAMA* 2013;309(6):570–7.
8. Mozaffarian D, Hao T, Rimm EB, Willett WC, Hu FB. Changes in diet and lifestyle and long-term weight gain in women and men. *N Engl J Med.* 2011;364(25):2392–404.
9. Duncan JL, Harrild KA, Iversen L, Lee AJ, Godden DJ. Long term outcomes in men screened for abdominal aortic aneurysm: prospective cohort study. *BMJ* 2012;344:e2958. doi:10.1136/bmj.e2958.
10. DuPont WD, Plummer WD. Power and sample size calculation. http://medipe.psu.ac.th/episoft/pssamplesize/. Accessed 19 May 2014.
11. Machin D, Campbell M, Tan SB, Tan SH. *Sample Size Tables for Clinical Studies.* Wiley-Blackwell. Third Edition (2009).
12. 5. Epi Info, Version 7. US Centers for Disease Control and Prevention. http://wwwn.cdc.gov/epiinfo/7/. Accessed 19 May 2014.
13. MRC Vitamin Study Research Group. Prevention of neural tube defects: result of the Medical Research Council Vitamin Study *Lancet* 1991 338 (8760):131–7.

CHAPTER 8

Quality of care studies

Chapters 5–7 focussed on studies that examined the relationship between exposures and outcome measures, usually for a well-defined clinical disorder. In a similar way, it is possible to examine experiences and attitudes of a specified group of people.

8.1 Purpose

Quality of care studies include either patients or health professionals or occasionally both, with the following general objectives:
- To examine patient satisfaction or experiences with a clinical service
- To evaluate a hospital/clinic system, or treatment or care pathway, by examining the experiences of both patients and health professionals
- Assessment of delivery of services by health professionals (e.g. nurses and doctors)
- To examine the impact of a service on clinical outcomes using the perspectives of both patients and clinicians
- To identify problems in a treatment or care pathway, make changes, and then assess the impact of the change

Many of these studies have the ultimate aim of making recommendations for improvement, or sometimes for further studies. Researchers often make the evaluation in their own institution, where the potential for change is greater, rather than regional or national recommendations, though others can use the findings and consider whether they could apply elsewhere. Quality of care studies are a major feature of **health services research**. Further details, including guidelines on how to report such studies, can be found elsewhere [1–4].

8.2 Design

There is a wide variety of designs, including qualitative studies (see page 12), but perhaps, the most common is the cross-sectional study (Chapter 5). They are often quick to undertake (<1 year) and can be conducted in a

A Concise Guide to Observational Studies in Healthcare, First Edition. Allan Hackshaw.

Box 8.1 Some key considerations when designing quality of care studies

Conduct
• Clear justification for the study: why the study is needed (e.g. a local issue that led to the study, or replication of other studies in a similar setting)
• If the study involves several departments within a hospital or several hospitals, support should be obtained upfront from a clinical lead in each unit (e.g. clinician or nurse), who could be made a project collaborator. This will help gaining access to staff (if the study is based on health professionals) or patients within those departments
• Response rate can be maximised by using simple and concise self-completed questionnaires, or face-to-face interviews in the clinic
• Anonymity should be assured in most studies, so that patients will not think their standard of care might be affected by their responses. Anonymity would not be required if patients are to be followed up and so needs to be tracked (e.g. changing health service delivery)

Outcomes
• It might be worth testing the questionnaire on a few patients first, to ensure that it will be interpreted correctly. Established questionnaires may need translating, and the phrases might be interpreted differently in different populations. Questionnaires developed specifically for the study might need testing and validation, unless the questions are simple and obvious
• Given the type of endpoints used (e.g. psychometric assessments) there could be much variability between participants, which can affect the quantitative results (e.g. wide 95% CIs and less reliable conclusions); therefore a larger study will be better than a small one

Potential bias
• Researchers should be aware of potential reporting bias, e.g. patients with bad experiences might be more likely to participate, and this will bias the results
• It should be made clear who conducted the study, and who had access to the patients, i.e. whether or not the study researchers work in the department or service being assessed
• Potential researcher bias, in that they use questions or influence interviews to produce the results they wanted
• Participants should be representative of the target population of interest, and so all should be approached, or a subset chosen by random sampling

Expected impact
• Researchers should indicate what sort of changes could be made to their health service, given the study findings
• If the study will compare changes in service delivery, it must be clearly specified which measures will be used before and after implementation, and the timeframe

single centre or a few centres (usually hospitals or general practice/family physician units).

As with all observational studies, specifying the sampling frame is essential, but this can often be relatively easy to do in quality of care studies, for example, all patients attending an emergency department January to June 2012, or all patients being treated for diabetes on a particular clinic list.

There are several key aspects to the design and conduct (Box 8.1).

8.3 Measuring variables

Unlike the observational studies in previous chapters, which had relatively well-defined exposures and outcomes, in quality of care studies, many factors are psychometric measures, based on perceived experiences, and these can be difficult to assess. They require patients or health professionals to consider many features of the health service of interest, and some of these features are likely to be correlated. Therefore, attempting to find specific reasons for poor satisfaction, or why certain services perform well (or badly), is not usually straightforward.

All measures associated with quality of care studies, except qualitative research, fall into one of the three categories: 'counting people', 'taking measurements on people', and time-to-event, though the latter is the least common.

Carefully structured questionnaires are essential to the success of quality of care studies and to obtain accurate data. While open-ended questions may be useful in eliciting general comments from the participants or finding information not previously known, it is best to have mostly questions requiring fixed responses. A **Likert-type scale** is commonly used, where the participant ticks one of several options in response to a statement. For example:

'I did not have to wait long before being seen by a doctor'
1. Strongly disagree
2. Disagree
3. Neither agree nor disagree
4. Agree
5. Strongly agree

Other options for response, depending on the type of statement, could be:
- Not important, somewhat important, very important, or essential
- Never, rarely, sometimes, most of the time, or always

This type of outcome can be analysed as 'counting people' endpoints (categorical data). Each item can be analysed separately, and the percentage of individuals can be reported in each group. Alternatively, focus could be on the extremes, whereby categories are combined (1+2 vs. 3+4+5, or 1+2+3 vs. 4+5), which creates a binary measure. Responses from several items could be combined (e.g. simply summed) and converted into a score (as with quality of life measures used in Section 5.9) to create a continuous measure. Another type of continuous measure involves asking people to indicate their response on a visual analogue scale (0–1 or 0–100, e.g. 0 = worst experience and 1 = best experience). All of these approaches can be analysed using methods presented in Chapters 2 to 4 if describing a single group of participants, or looking at associations among them.

If developing a study-specific questionnaire, items should not be repetitive, that is, asking the same thing in slightly different ways. Also, the layout and format of a self-completed questionnaire should be attractive, with sufficient space between questions to avoid the text looking cramped on the page. A poorly laid out questionnaire can make it difficult to complete, and so lead to lower response rate or missing data.

8.4 Collecting the data

Data are often obtained directly from the participants (patients or health professionals), using self-completed questionnaires or interviews.

Questionnaires that have already been developed can be obtained from the published literature and the internet, but researchers may also develop their own, to tailor it to their specific institution, and so bring out key features that led to the research project. Self-completed questionnaires have the advantage that they can be sent to a larger number of people and can cover a wider range of topics, but the main limitation is a potentially low response rate.

Alternatively, face-to-face interviews can encourage participation, reduce the non-response rate, and minimise missing data, but require staff to undertake them. This may involve training, which is particularly important when dealing with psychometric measures and the potential for interviewer bias (see Box 1.6). When quality of care studies are conducted in a specific hospital department, patients could be asked to complete the questionnaire while waiting to see the health professional or afterwards.

8.5 Sample size

Study size is often limited by the size of the available sampling frame, for example, the number of stroke patients on an outpatient list. Also, the desired length of the study will have an effect, because if it might take 5 years to accrue a specified study size, the researchers may need to consider whether or not to proceed. However, quality of care studies are often exploratory, so in general, the more participants, the better.

It is possible to specify an important endpoint and calculate a sample size using the same method as for cross-sectional studies (Box 5.8); See Examples 1 and 2.

8.6 Analysing data

The main results of quality of care studies tend to be descriptive, but additional analyses can examine associations (e.g. differences between males and females, or seniority of staff), and the methods of analyses are the same as those in Chapter 3 (effect sizes, 95% confidence intervals (CIs) and p-values).

Although many of the outcomes (e.g. psychometric measures) are different to clinical or physiological outcomes presented in previous chapters, the statistical methods in Chapters 2 and 3 still apply (particularly linear and logistic regression). Other analyses could involve obtaining **correlation coefficients** between two continuous factors (to quantify the relationship), measures of agreement between people or techniques that measure the same outcome (**Bland–Altman statistic** or **Kappa statistic**), or multivariate methods such as **principal components** or **factor analysis** (which are often exploratory analyses that aim to reduce a large number of factors to a few dimensions) [5].

8.7 Example 1: patient satisfaction with a service

Box 8.2 [6] is an example of a common type of quality of care study, focussing on a single department within a single clinic (quality of emergency care). The study took only 1 month to complete. The researchers provided a sample size calculation assuming 63% of patients would have 'favourable experiences', and the 95% CI width was required to be ±3%, yielding a target sample size of 995 (Box 5.9).

Box 8.2 Example 1: Quality of care [6]

Objective: To examine the quality of care among patients visiting an emergency care clinic.

Location: An emergency department in a single clinic in Ethiopia (tertiary/referral centre).

Study participants: 963 patients attending the clinic in May 2012.

Design: The hospital has five emergency suites (adults and children). Every fourth patient on the list from each suite was asked to participate (a form of random sampling), during both day and night. If the patient was unable to participate due to distress (or too young), the person accompanying them was asked to take part. Patients (or their companion) were approached as they were leaving the clinic. Those who accepted were interviewed face-to-face in a private area by a nurse, health officer, or health technician who did not work in the emergency department, and had received training on how to perform the interviews.

Outcomes: Quality of care was measured using a standard questionnaire (Press Ganey). 'Quality of emergency care' was addressed by perceived satisfaction of care, using patient satisfaction defined as feelings of pleasure or disappointment with the service. 'Patient satisfaction' was measured using 20 questions, each with a Likert scale (five options). The questionnaires were tested on 20 patients before starting the main study, and changes made so that the questions were suitable to this particular group.

Results: Figure 8.1 and Table 8.1.

Authors' conclusion: There is a low level of patient satisfaction related to several aspects of the service in the emergency department. It is important to revise the service delivery to improve staff courtesy and reduce discrimination, at all points of care to increase patient satisfaction.

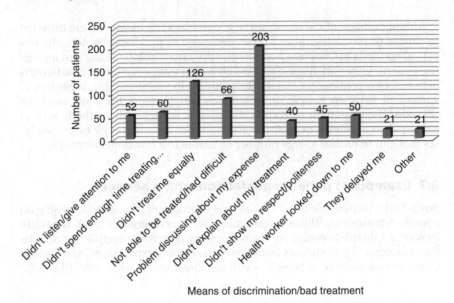

Means of discrimination/bad treatment

Figure 8.1 Bar chart showing perceived reasons for discrimination or being treated badly among 706 patients out of the 963 in the study in Box 8.1 who reported this experience. The figure shows the absolute number of patients on the y-axis, but it is better to show percentages, for example, 'Didn't treat me equally' would be 17.8% (126/706), and 'Problem discussing about my expense' would be 28.7% (203/706). Source: Taye et al. 2014 [6]. Originally published by BioMed Central.

Table 8.1 Selected results from the study in Box 8.2.

Four items from the 20-item questionnaire	Level of satisfaction and numeric score				
	Very dissatisfied 1 % (n)	Dissatisfied 2 % (n)	Fair 3 % (n)	Satisfied 4 % (n)	Very satisfied 5 % (n)
Comfort of the waiting area	3.6 (35)	19.2 (185)	27.9 (269)	41.3 (398)	7.9 (76)
Information given about medications	10.6 (102)	25.6 (247)	28.0 (270)	31.0 (299)	4.7 (45)
Amount of time spent with the health professional	2.5 (24)	10.2 (97)	26.8 (258)	48.3 (465)	12.4 (119)
Overall cleanliness of the hospital	5.3 (51)	16.5 (159)	21.7 (209)	45.9 (442)	10.6 (102)

There were 963 patients, so fthe numbers in brackets should sum to this in each row, and the percentages sum to 100.

Response rate

It is important to know the available number of participants from the sampling frame, so that the response rate (the number who took part divided by the total number available or approached) can be obtained. The response rate in the example was reported to be very high, 96.8%, and this may have been due to the research team physically approaching the patients as they were leaving the emergency unit and interviewing them, instead of giving them a self-completed questionnaire.

Results

As with all descriptive studies, there should be a simple summary table showing the main characteristics of the participants, and this was provided in the paper. It showed the number and percentage of the recruited 963 patients according to age group, sex, residence, occupation, day of visit, time of day of arrival, and emergency suite visited. There was also a bar chart showing the distribution of patients according to type of diagnosis.

The 20-item survey was summarised in a table showing percentages for each item according to each of the five possible responses (Table 8.1). This is a simple way to show the results for multiple categorical measures. For example, it is easy to see with which features patients were most satisfied (e.g. amount of time spent with the health professional), and those with the least satisfaction (e.g. information given about medications), just by examining the size of the percentages.

Some researchers treat this type of categorical factor as if it were continuous and report the means (the average of the numeric scores 1–5 among the patients) and standard deviations. For example, in this study, the mean score for 'amount of time spent with the health professional' was 3.58, with standard deviation 0.92. Although, this might give a general idea about the results of a factor there are problems:

- The mean score does not have any clinical meaning; the numbers 1–5 are labels for qualitative responses, there is no real numeric unit of measurement.
- It assumes a quantitative relationship between the responses, for example, that a score of 4 is twice as big as a score of 2, but given that 4 = satisfied and 2 = dissatisfied, we cannot determine that one category is associated with twice the amount of satisfaction in relation to the other.
- Mean scores can mask (dilute) differences between groups, whereas the percentage with extreme scores ('very dissatisfied' or 'very satisfied') could give a clearer picture of the results.

One specific item was whether the patients had experienced discrimination or were treated badly, and 73.3% (706/963) said that they had. Figure 8.1, a bar chart showing the perceived reasons, is a clear way to present this type of data.

Multivariable logistic regression was also used to examine relationships between satisfaction/no satisfaction (outcome measure) and several factors. For example, those attending on Friday were twice as likely to be satisfied as those attending on Sunday, adjusted odds ratio 1.9, 95% CI 1.1–1.3.

Another result provided in the paper was **Cronbach's alpha** [7], which is a measure of internal consistency among the 20 items on the questionnaire, that is, how closely related a set of items are as a group. The items should all be measuring the same (similar thing), that is, patient satisfaction, so they should be correlated. Cronbach's alpha is a coefficient, considered to be a measure of reliability or consistency. The value is 0 to 1, and high values indicate high internal consistency and provide evidence that the items measure an underlying construct. In the study, Cronbach's alpha was 0.88, which is high.

How good is the evidence?
The study was conducted to provide, for the first time in the region, evidence on patient care in an emergency clinic, for the Ministry of Health.

Some strengths and limitations were:
• Use of a validated questionnaire.
• The questionnaire was originally in English, but after being translated to the local language (Amharic), it was back-translated to English by a different person, to check that the translation was accurate. This is a valuable process when using surveys written in another language, though there is sometimes a financial cost to this.
• Patients were approached at any time of the day and randomly selected, so the group who participated should be representative of all those attending the emergency department.
• The interviewers did not work in the department, thus minimising or avoiding interviewer bias.
• The high response rate should mean that the findings are generalisable to the population seen in this hospital.
• Patients were only recruited in 1 month of the year (May), and experiences may be better or worse at other times.
• The study was only conducted in a single referral hospital, so it may not be generalisable to other types of hospitals elsewhere in the country.

The researchers were able to identify specific points of care in the emergency department and so make clear recommendations.

8.8 Example 2: patient satisfaction with treatment

This example (Box 8.3) [8] was based on a study to examine how satisfied patients were with their current treatment, in this case warfarin. It also aimed to determine how willing they were to change to an alternative drug (dabigatran), which is just as effective but has other benefits (fewer follow-up clinic visits required, and patients can drink alcohol while on therapy). The sample size was based on requiring a 90% CI to be ±5% for a response rate of 50% (Box 5.8).

Response rate
It was not stated how many patients were listed on the anticoagulant clinic list, but it is useful to know that consecutive patients were approached (i.e. specific patients were not targeted); 273 were asked to participate, of whom 260 accepted, a response rate of 95%, which is high.

Box 8.3 Example 2: patient satisfaction with treatment [8]

Objective: To evaluate patient satisfaction with their current warfarin treatment and obtain their opinion on switching to another drug.

Location: A single anticoagulant clinic in Georgia, US.

Study participants: 260 patients currently on warfarin, who attended their usual clinic visit in March 2011–March 2012.

Design: The target sample size was 260, and consecutive patients seen in the clinic were asked to participate until this number was reached. All 260 patients were given a survey asking about their satisfaction with warfarin. Those with non-valvular atrial fibrillation (n = 130) were also asked to complete a section about changing therapy from warfarin to a new drug (dabigatran). The full survey (both sections) could be completed in about 5 minutes, and when finished, patients put it into a drop box in the clinic.

Outcomes: The self-completed questionnaire was developed specifically for the study and contained 15 questions; 14 were based on a Likert-type scale (five responses), and the other asked about how much more the patient would pay for the new drug (five categories). It appears that the name (dabigatran) was not mentioned on the questionnaire; patients were just made aware of a new licensed drug. There was no mention of whether the questionnaire had been tested on patients first or validated.

Results: Table 8.2.

Authors' conclusion: Patients are generally satisfied with warfarin but willing to consider a new drug; however, the cost of the drug is the major barrier to switching.

Results

As with Example 1, a summary table showing the main characteristics of the participants (e.g. age, sex, ethnic background) was included in the published paper.

Patients had to respond to questions about their use of warfarin, as well as attributes of a new drug, illustrating the relatively complex thought processes that may be required of patients in studies like these. Table 8.2 shows selected results, from which it can be concluded that:

- Patients were very familiar with using warfarin (81.8% scored 5).
- Patients were dissatisfied about having to moderate their alcohol intake, due to the interaction between alcohol and warfarin (55.3% scored 1).
- Many seem to prefer fewer clinic visits associated with dabigatran (40.5% scored 5).
- The cost of dabigatran would put many people off switching (31.4% scored 1).
- Patients were seen in all five categories of each item; so not all patients were bothered by the issue of alcohol (15.0% scored 5), and several would not mind paying more per month (15.7% scored 5).

How good is the evidence?

Some characteristics of the study patients were as follows: 45.1% males, 40.7% African-American, 24.1% aged >70, 59.2% educated up to high school only, and 19.4% employed. These are likely to be different from many other clinics,

Table 8.2 Selected results from the study in Box 8.3.

Questions (some rephrased from original survey to be concise here)	Response (% of individuals)*					
	1	2	3	4	5	N/A
How confident are you about handling of your warfarin treatment?	2.4	0.8	2.4	9.1	81.8	3.6
How much does warfarin limit the alcoholic beverage you might wish to drink?	55.3	6.7	7.9	4.0	15.0	11.1
Overall, how much are you satisfied with your warfarin treatment?	2.4	0.4	4.0	11.1	77.9	4.3
If you knew there was a new oral anticoagulant medication that is as effective as warfarin in preventing strokes, would you be willing to change to the new medication?	9.9	7.4	20.7	13.2	37.2	11.6
If you know that this new medication requires less frequent follow-up visits, would you be willing to change?	9.9	6.6	9.1	24.0	40.5	9.9
Would you be willing to change to the new medication if it costs you more per month?	31.4	15.7	18.2	9.9	15.7	9.1

*The response to each item is on a 1–5 scale, where:
1 = least favourable or satisfied, or strongly disagree.
5 = most favourable or satisfied, or strongly agree.
N/A = not answered, (i.e. missing or incomplete data).

and therefore some results may not be generalisable, although the findings on willingness to pay for the new drug were considered to apply to patients with similar characteristics elsewhere. If the ultimate purpose of the study was to make recommendations only for patients in this clinic, the researchers have probably gathered enough evidence to attempt to change practice locally.

Some strengths and limitations were:
• Patients needed to balance several advantages and disadvantages of both the current and new medications, with few details given about the new drug, all done within a short questionnaire.
• The purpose seemed to be to obtain an initial assessment from patients, and a short questionnaire maximised response.
• Several patients did not complete certain questions, for example, 3.6% did not answer the question about their confidence in using warfarin, while 11.1% did not provide a response to the question on alcohol. Some consideration of possible responder bias might be useful.

8.9 Example 3: assessing a service and improving service delivery

This example (Box 8.4) [9] was based on a study to estimate adherence to treatment among patients who had had a renal transplant, which factors influence it, and whether adherence could be improved. It therefore had two

Box 8.4 Example 3: Examining adherence to treatment and improving service delivery [9]

Objective: To examine non-adherence to treatment among patients who had a renal transplant and to evaluate whether more intense clinical monitoring and reduced pill number could increase adherence.

Location: A single outpatient clinic in Naples, Italy.

Study participants: 310 patients who were attending the outpatient clinic and were aged >18, had their renal transplant >1 year ago, had no cognitive impairment and were able to read and understand the questionnaire. All eligible patients within an 8-month period were approached.

Design: A cross-sectional and prospective cohort study. All 310 patients were asked to complete 3 questionnaires at baseline. Then the 160 who were taking twice-daily tacrolimus were asked if they would switch to a once-daily formulation (same total dose), of whom 121 accepted and 39 declined. In addition, there were 150 patients who were on cyclosporine. All patients were given the same questionnaires after 3 and 6 months, during their usual clinic visit.

Outcomes: Two questionnaires were based on a Transplant Learning Centre programme, with Likert-type scales (0–5 for each question), and measured quality of life, patient satisfaction, and their views on the care they receive. The scores were summed over the questions to produce a Life Satisfaction Index and a Transplant Care Index. The third questionnaire (Immunosuppressant Therapy Adherence Scale (ITAS)) measured adherence to treatment using several questions (0–4 for each question), which were summed to produce an adherence score (≤ 10 non-adherence, >10 adherence).

Results: Table 8.3 and Figure 8.2.

Authors' conclusion: The prevalence of non-adherence was high and associated with life satisfaction and anxiety. Reducing the number of pills taken daily increases adherence.

designs: cross-sectional (for the descriptive aims) and prospective cohort (to observe changes in adherence over time).

Response rate
All renal transplant patients who attended the outpatient clinic during an 8-month period were approached; 347 were invited, of whom 310 agreed to take part, a response rate of 89%, which is acceptably high.

Results
As with the previous two examples, there was a table in the published paper summarising the patient characteristics (e.g. age, sex, blood pressure, body mass index, and standard laboratory tests such as haemoglobin).

The proportion of patients classified by the researchers as being non-adherent was 23.5% (73/310); the definition of non-adherence was having an ITAS score ≤ 10 (range 0–12). However, among the 73 patients who were non-adherent, 54 had a score of exactly 10, and 19 had ≤ 9. Clearly, the prevalence

Table 8.3 Selected measures of life satisfaction and quality of care from the example in Box 8.4.

Item	Mean score (standard deviation)		p-value
	Adherent patients (n = 237)	Non-adherent patients (n = 73)	
Relationship with medical care	3.91 (0.43)	3.49 (0.61)	0.0007
Satisfaction with health care	3.84 (0.41)	3.72 (0.55)	0.04
Life in general	3.45 (0.77)	3.04 (0.60)	0.0002
Keeping scheduled follow-up	3.86 (0.39)	3.50 (0.85)	0.0006

Each item is on a scale 0–4, where 0 = poor conditions and 4 = best conditions.

of non-adherence will change with different score cut-offs. Other researchers have recommended a cut-off of ≤9, which could have been a more objectively chosen value for the study used in this example (i.e. selected independently of the researchers and the results), yielding a prevalence of non-adherence of only 6.1%. Nevertheless, a breakdown of the scores is helpful for readers.

Table 8.3 is based on the cross-sectional study and compares selected outcomes between those classified as adherent and non-adherent. It suggests that patients who were adherent had a better relationship with medical staff, were more satisfied with the care they received, happier about life in general, and more likely to keep to the scheduled clinic visits. However, as discussed in Example 1, the analysis is based on treating the scores (0–4) as if they were a continuous measure, which may not be appropriate, so the reliability of the p-value is questionable. Comparing the proportion in the lowest categories (e.g. 0 + 1) or the highest (e.g. 3 + 4) would have been better and clearer. Nevertheless, the table provides an approximate idea of the differences between the two patient groups.

The main result from the cohort stage of the study is shown in Figure 8.2, in which the prevalence of non-adherence decreased from 23.5 (T0) to 15% (T6) in the shift group. A p-value of <0.05 is indicated, but it is not clear whether the statistical test used was a standard chi-square test, which will assume that the patients at 6 months are different from those at baseline. The correct test in this situation is a McNemar's test, which only compares patients who had discordant results, that is, those who were adherent at baseline and then became non-adherent versus those who were non-adherent at baseline and then became adherent [5].

How good is the evidence?
The study allowed a description of adherence in this particular patient population and also how it can be improved.

Some strengths and limitations were:
- All consecutive patients seen in the clinic were approached.
- Several outcomes were assessed, including patient satisfaction with the care they receive and measures of well-being.

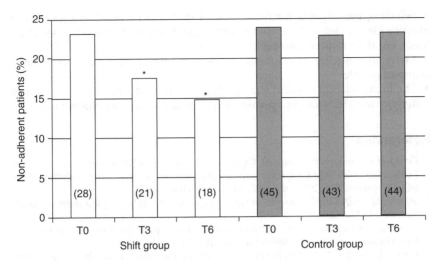

Figure 8.2 Prevalence of non-adherence to treatment among patients who switched from twice-daily drug (tacrolimus) to once daily (shift group) or those on cyclosporine or refused to switch (control group). T0 is baseline, and T3 and T6 are 3 and 6 months later, respectively. *p-value < 0.05, compared with the baseline value. Source: Sabbatini et al. 2014 [9]. Reproduced by permission of Dove Medical Press Ltd.

- Patients in the control group (who did not switch treatment) consisted of two distinct types: those who were not taking the drug of interest (tacrolimus) and those who were on tacrolimus but declined to switch to the once-daily therapy. Therefore, the group who did switch and the controls are probably not comparable. However, the data do suggest that once-daily therapy could improve compliance.
- It is not known whether long-term adherence improvement remains the same after 6 months.

These findings could be used by medical staff to provide more attention to particular patients and discuss issues over the importance of treatment, as well as try to improve their well-being. The ultimate aim was to increase the chance that the transplant remains successful, if treatment compliance is maximised.

8.10 Key points

- There is a wide variety of quality of care studies, with cross-sectional designs being one of the most common.
- Outcome measures tend to be based on psychometric questionnaires (self-completed or face-to-face interviews).
- Questions with fixed responses (Likert-type scales) are generally preferred, compared with open-ended questions.

- Selecting participants for these studies (patients or health professionals) must be clearly defined (sampling frame, eligibility, and method of selecting them, i.e. all or random sample).
- Many analyses are descriptive, summarising the characteristics of a single group of people.
- The interpretation of effect sizes such as relative risk, odds ratio, and mean difference (and 95% CIs and p-values) is the same as in other chapters.

References

1. Davidoff F, Batalden P, Stevens D, Ogrinc G, Mooney SE; SQUIRE development group. Publication guidelines for quality improvement studies in health care: evolution of the SQUIRE project. BMJ 2009;338:a3152. doi: 10.1136/bmj.a3152.
2. Standards for QUality Improvement Reporting Excellence. http://squire-statement.org/. Accessed 16 May 2014.
3. Baker GR. Strengthening the contribution of quality improvement research to evidence based health care. Qual Saf Health Care 2006;15:150–1.
4. Lynn J, Baily MA, Bottrell M, Jennings B, Levine RJ, Davidoff F, et al. The ethics of using quality improvement methods in health care. Ann Intern Med 2007;146:666–73.
5. Kirkwood BR, Sterne JAC. Essential Medical Statistics. Blackwell Science. Second Edition (2003).
6. Taye BW, Yassin MO, Kebede ZT. Quality of emergency medical care in Gondar University Referral Hospital, Northwest Ethiopia: a survey of patients' perspectives. BMC Emerg Med 2014;14(1):2.
7. Bland JM, Altman DG. Cronbach's alpha. BMJ 1997;314:572.
8. Elewa HF, Deremer CE, Keller K, Gujral J, Joshua TV. Patients satisfaction with warfarin and willingness to switch to dabigatran: a patient survey. J Thromb Thrombolysis 2013; doi 10.1007/s11239-013-0976-y.
9. Sabbatini M, Garofalo G, Borrelli S, Vitale S, Torino M, Capone D, et al. Efficacy of a reduced pill burden on therapeutic adherence to calcineurin inhibitors in renal transplant recipients: an observational study. Patient Prefer Adherence 2014;8:73–81.

CHAPTER 9

Prognostic markers for predicting outcomes

Many observational studies aim to examine the association between an exposure and outcome. A special case of this is to develop a model using various characteristics to predict whether someone is likely to have or develop a specified outcome or not. Prognostic marker research involves some of the analytical methods used in previous chapters, but there are additional concepts. The approaches covered in this chapter can be used to examine screening and diagnostic tests. Studies using genetic prognostic markers are becoming increasingly common, and these also have some special considerations.

9.1 Prognostic markers and models

The main purpose of a **prognostic marker** or model (the **exposure**) is to try to predict the outcome for an individual.[#] The marker could be a simple features such as age and gender, a clinical measurement such as blood pressure, imaging markers (from X-rays, MRI, or CT scans), or a biological marker or genetic factor measured in the blood, urine, or tissue. (All types of these markers are used as examples in this chapter.) The outcome could be the occurrence of a new disorder in an unaffected person, disease progression or death for a person who is already ill, or any well-defined change in health status. In practice, only **diagnostic markers** (or tests) are designed to show whether or not an individual will have a specific outcome (with almost complete certainty), so prognostic markers and models essentially estimate the risk (chance) of the outcome. The clinical value of a good prognostic factor is that it can identify people (or patients) who are likely to benefit from an intervention, and thus prevent an adverse outcome, or it identifies people appropriate for a diagnostic test, which is too harmful or expensive to give to everyone.

Several aspects (Box 9.1) need to be considered when proposing a prognostic marker (or model), in addition to the quantitative measures that are

---

[#] In this sense, the term **predictive marker** might seem more appropriate than **prognostic marker**, but the former is commonly understood to specifically relate to markers that forecast ('predict') outcomes *after people have received a certain intervention*.

A Concise Guide to Observational Studies in Healthcare, First Edition. Allan Hackshaw.

Box 9.1 What to consider when examining a prognostic marker (quantitative measures are described elsewhere in the chapter)

- How common is the disorder (or outcome)? If very rare, applying the marker to everyone might not be worthwhile.
- How easy is it to measure the marker?
- Is the marker reliably measured? Only properly validated biomarkers should be used, and assays that are commercially available does not necessarily mean that they measure what they are supposed to.
- What is the extent of measurement error? This can be minimised by central reviews of scans/images, good sample collection processes using a standard operating procedure, or central laboratory analyses with good quality control systems.
- Financial costs of measuring the marker (e.g. cost of scans or cost of obtaining and processing biological samples)?
- What happens to people who are classified as marker positive, for example, additional tests or treatments? Are these tests or interventions harmful or expensive?
- Being aware that a prognostic model (particularly if based on several factors) may need to be updated over time.

---

described in the following sections. More details are provided in a BMJ series [1–4] and elsewhere [5–7].

9.2 Study design

Prognostic markers can be examined using the designs covered in Chapters 5–7. The preferred design is a cohort study, ideally prospective, although retrospective studies could be acceptable (acknowledging issues over missing data). This is because absolute risk, given the marker result, can be estimated in a cohort study, but it is not possible to do this in a case–control study, where the number of cases and controls is chosen by the researcher. However, it is possible to obtain information on prognostic performance from a case–control study (e.g. by mathematical modelling) and apply it to the background risk for a disorder. This needs to be done carefully, ensuring that both the cases and controls come from the target population of interest. Other types of studies include those based on patient records, which are likely to have issues over missing data, and quality of data, so the conclusions of these are often to recommend further prospective studies to confirm the findings.

Measuring prognostic performance

There are two useful statistical considerations when examining prognostic markers: **effect sizes** and **prognostic performance**. Effect sizes are measures of association, such as relative risk and odds or hazard ratio (Chapter 3). They

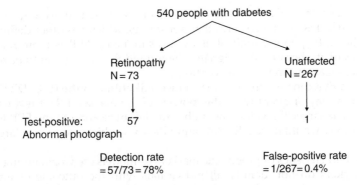

Figure 9.1 Illustration of measures of prognostic performance using a study of people with insulin-dependent diabetes, in which the prognostic marker (or screening test) is a retinal photograph of the eye (abnormal or normal). The sensitivity is also 78%, and the specificity would be 99.6% (1 − FPR).

indicate whether the relationship between a marker and a disorder is small, moderate or large. Many researchers only provide effect sizes when they report prognostic studies, which is the first step, but these do not really tell us how good a prognostic marker is at forecasting outcomes. Both measures are ultimately required.

Prognostic performance is examined using two quantitative parameters: **detection rate** (**DR**, also called **sensitivity** or **true positive rate**) and **false-positive rate** (**FPR**, which is 1 − **specificity**). These are illustrated in Figure 9.1.

Unlike effect sizes, which are calculated by analysing all individuals together, DR and FPR always consider them as two separate groups: people with the outcome (affected) and those without (unaffected).

It is important to have both the DR and FPR. A high DR (e.g. 85%) is meaningless without knowing whether the FPR is low or high (e.g. 5 or 50%). A diagnostic marker or test should have a DR close to 100% and FPR close to 0%. There is no gold standard for what makes a good prognostic marker, in terms of size of DR and FPR. Figure 9.1 shows an excellent marker (high DR and very low FPR), but many other markers have lower DRs (50–70%) and higher FPRs (e.g. 5–20%).

Marker performance can be considered in relation to the seriousness of the disorder, and what happens to people who have positive test results. For example, markers for predicting Down's syndrome in pregnancy have a DR of 70–85%, but this comes from specifying a low FPR (<5%), because women who are test positive are offered an invasive and expensive diagnostic test (e.g. amniocentesis), which has a risk of miscarriage. In contrast, mean corpuscular haemoglobin is used to screen for β-thalassaemia in pregnancy and because the aim is to detect almost all cases (DR close to 100%), the FPR can be relatively high (up to 37%) The subsequent test is only another blood (diagnostic) test that, although relatively expensive, is not harmful.

The most commonly used terms in the literature are sensitivity and specificity, although DR is a better term than sensitivity, which has other definitions in medicine (e.g. lower limit of assay measurement). FPR is more relevant than specificity, because it designates the individuals who go on to have further investigations and/or interventions.

DR and FPR can be combined to produce a **likelihood ratio** (LR = DR/FPR), which is a way of quantifying the 'power' of the marker. LR = 1 is a useless marker. The larger the value, the higher the DR in relation to the FPR (e.g. a good marker would have DR = 80% and FPR = 5%, which produces a large LR of 16).

Two characteristics of prognostic markers or models are worth noting:
1. Markers do not identify <u>all</u> individuals with the outcome of interest (cases are always missed), that is, DR would never be 100%.
2. Markers will always pick up individuals without the outcome ('error' and these individuals could have unnecessary further investigations or interventions): that is the FPR would always exceed 0.

Although DR and FPR are important parameters, it is also necessary to see how well the marker works in the population of interest. This is achieved by examining the **odds of being affected given a positive result** (OAPR) or **positive predictive value** (PPV); see example 9.1 (page 177).

When several prognostic markers are examined together, they should be combined into a model using multivariable linear, logistic, or Cox regressions depending on whether the outcome measure involves 'taking measurements on people', 'counting people', or measuring the time until an event occurs.

Effect sizes such as relative risk, odds ratio, and hazard ratio measure the relationship between an exposure (prognostic marker) and outcome. This is conceptually different from the prognostic performance of the marker, which examines how well it predicts the outcome. It is not commonly recognised that a prognostic marker needs to be very strongly associated with the disorder (i.e. high or low odds or hazard ratios) to have a good performance [8]. For example, maternal serum alpha-fetoprotein (AFP) is a prognostic marker for neural tube defects in pregnancy (and used for prenatal screening). The odds ratio between the highest and lowest quintile of AFP is 246 (a very large effect), and the corresponding DR = 91% and FPR = 5% indicates good performance. In comparison, although the association between serum cholesterol and ischaemic heart disease is established and appears to be a large effect (odds ratio of 2.7 between the highest and lowest quintiles among UK men), the DR is only 15% for a FPR of 5%; that is, cholesterol is not an effective prognostic marker, because it has a poor performance [8]. Having a moderate or reasonably strong association does not necessarily mean that the marker is good at predicting outcomes.

Training and validation datasets (examining several markers)
When using a single prognostic marker, one dataset is often sufficient when the cut-points used to estimate DR and FPR are already pre-established and have not been developed by the researchers. For example, in Figure 9.1, the

retinal photograph can only be normal or abnormal, and for a continuous marker like blood pressure, fixed values such as ≥ 120, ≥ 130, ≥ 140 mmHg, etc. can be used. Neither of these is driven by the actual dataset. However, if there is uncertainty over the generalisability of the study findings, then it might be appropriate to examine the marker in another (independent) dataset.

When examining several prognostic markers, each will probably have different units of measurement, so they need to be combined to produce a single measure, and then a cut-off point can be applied, as if dealing with a single marker. This combined measure and cut-off point come from a statistical model, and the model needs to be developed by the researchers. This could be done using a large study that is split into two, or two separate studies of similar individuals, so that the prognostic model is developed with one dataset (**training dataset**) and tested on another (**validation dataset**). Using the same dataset to both develop and test the model will give biased (optimistic) estimates of performance. The validation dataset can also be used to check whether the model is sufficiently reliable by comparing estimated (predicted) with observed risk values.

Splitting a dataset (half training and half validation or, two-thirds training and one-third validation) could be performed randomly, but then the two groups should be similar to each other, and this could overestimate prognostic performance. It is better to split the dataset using time (e.g. the first two-thirds of registered participants in the study form the training set, and the last third make up the validation set). This has the advantage of attempting to validate the model prospectively, which is similar to what would be done in practice (i.e. a model developed now, to be applied to future individuals). The number of events is as important as study size, so it may be better to divide the data according to events (see Example 3), to ensure that sufficient numbers of events occur in each dataset to produce reliable results. Having a completely independent dataset (as the validation data) is ideal because it will address generalisability, but it can often be difficult to find one that has similar individuals to the one used to develop the model and that has all the factors measured.

Other methods are **cross-validation** or **bootstrapping** (especially if the dataset is not large enough to be split). With cross-validation, one individual is removed, and the model is developed using the remaining individuals and then tested/validated on the removed individual, who is classified as marker positive or not. This is repeated for every individual in the dataset, and DR and FPR are obtained by counting the number of positives in the affected and unaffected groups. With bootstrapping, if there are, for example, 435 individuals in the study, a random sample of 435 is selected, after replacing each person (so an individual could be included several times in the sample or not at all). The model is developed on this sample and then tested on the original dataset. The process is repeated at least 100 times, with the average model performance estimated.

Another approach involves using the dataset to produce statistical parameters (e.g. means, standard deviations and correlation coefficients), that are incorporated into a model which produces DR, FPR and OAPR [9]. An advantage of these methods, over splitting the dataset, is that all of the data values are used to develop and test the model.

9.3 Sample size

Prognostic markers are often examined as part of translational sub-studies within an observational study that is already established (completed or ongoing). Therefore, an estimation of the sample size can be made to only check whether the study is large enough for the marker analysis.

A simple sample size for DR or FPR can be established by specifying the width of the 95% confidence intervals (CIs) that would be considered sufficiently narrow. This will depend on what is feasible and will involve guessing what the DRs and FPRs are likely to be. Table 9.1 illustrates this. Small sample sizes give wide intervals, and if researchers intend for the interval around either the DR or FPR to be fairly narrow, then large numbers are needed. A noticeable gain occurs in increasing the sample size from 50 to 200, but not from 400 to 1000.

When considering the sample size of a training dataset used for several prognostic markers examined together, there are no standard sample size methods for multivariable regression analysis. It is recommended that there should be at least 10 events per included marker [10]. If there are eight factors, therefore, ≥ 80 events are required, and the researchers must then scale up to the number of participants needed to achieve this.

For a single prognostic marker, only one sample size estimation may be needed, but for several markers, which involve separate training and validation datasets, a sample size could be calculated for each.

Table 9.1 95% CIs for varying DR (sensitivity) and FPR (1-specificity), according to the number of individuals available for each measure.

	Sample size used for either DR or FPR			
	$N=50$	$N=200$	$N=400$	$N=1000$
DR (%)				
60	46–73	53–67	55–65	57–63
70	57–83	64–76	66–74	67–73
80	69–91	74–85	76–84	77–82
90	82–98	86–94	87–92	88–92
FPR (%)				
5	0–11	2–8	3–7	4–6
10	2–18	6–14	7–13	8–12
15	5–25	10–20	11–18	13–17
20	9–31	14–25	16–24	17–22

For example, if DR = 60%, p = 0.60 and standard error (SE) is $\sqrt{p \times (1-p)/N}$. 95% CI is $p \pm 1.96 \times SE$.

9.4 Analysing data and interpreting results

Outcome measures based on 'counting people' (binary or categorical endpoints)

In the two examples below, the outcome is either a disorder (affected or unaffected) or mortality (dead or alive). Both are based on a single prognostic marker and so may only require a single dataset (not separate training and validation datasets), because the definition of marker positive is pre-defined.

Example 9.1 Head injury and cranial haematoma

This example is one in which the marker, like the outcome measure, is also a binary (categorical) factor. The study was based on people with a head injury, who attended accident and emergency departments at three hospitals [11]; those who felt disorientated were analysed separately from those who felt fine.[#] The prognostic marker was an X-ray, to look for the presence or absence of a skull fracture, and the outcome measure was having a cranial haematoma following a head injury. The researchers examined medical records from 545 patients with a haematoma, and 2773 who did not. Because this was not a prospective study (it had a case–control design), the results in the unaffected patients were applied to all admissions to the three hospitals to create results as if they came from a prospective study. Table 9.2 shows the main findings.

The table illustrates what all prognostic markers do: they change a person's risk. Before the patients with a head injury, who were not disorientated, had an X-ray, their risk was 0.05% (the background or overall risk). After the marker result is known, the risk either reduces (to 0.02% for marker negative patients, no skull fracture) or increases (to 3.1% for marker-positive patients, with skull fracture). The risk in the marker-positive group is sometimes called PPV, or OAPR.

For patients who are not disorientated, the odds ratio[#] for having a haematoma (skull fracture vs. no fracture) is 191. The corresponding relative risk is 185 (55/55 + 1721 ÷ 29/29 + 173486), close to the OR. This is a huge effect (strong association), which has a good prognostic performance: DR = 65% (65% of those with a haematoma had a skull fracture) and FPR = 1% (only 1% of those without a haematoma had a skull fracture). The OAPR is the risk of having the disorder (here, a haematoma) only among those who are marker positive (here, skull fracture). It is 1:31 (or absolute risk of 3.1%, PPV). This means that to detect one affected case, 31 patients without a haematoma need to be followed up and investigated (hospital admissions and CT scans) unnecessarily. (Alternatively, only 3.1% of orientated people with a skull fracture have a haematoma.) Therefore, although this marker itself has a strong association with having a haematoma it is not very efficient *when used to predict a haematoma in a population*. The problem is not the marker; it is the

---

[#] In fact, being disorientated is another prognostic factor, but in this example, it is not combined with the skull X-ray by analysing all patients together.

[#] OR is used more often than relative risk, because it is produced by regression analyses when evaluating several markers together.

Table 9.2 Findings from a study examining the performance of a prognostic marker (skull X-ray) in predicting the presence or absence of a cranial haematoma in patients with a head injury.

	Not disorientated			Disorientated		
	Haematoma	Unaffected	Absolute risk (%)	Haematoma	Unaffected	Absolute risk (%)
Fracture	55	1,721	3.1 (PPV)	357	1,214	22.7 (PPV)
No fracture	29	173,486	0.02	104	12,466	0.83
Total	84	175,207	0.05	461	13,680	3.3
	DR=65%	FPR=1%		DR=77%	FPR=9%	
		LR=65			LR=8.5	
Odds ratio (95% CI)	191 (122–300)			35 (28–44)		

DR, detection rate; FPR, false-positive rate; LR, likelihood ratio; DR÷FPR.
Odds ratio: odds of having a haematoma in those with a fracture compared with those without a fracture.

DR for haematoma is found from the number with a fracture/the total in the column (e.g. 65% =55/84). Similarly for FPR (1% = 1721 / 175, 207).
The absolute risk for having a haematoma is the number affected divided by the total in the row. For example, 3.1% is 55/(55 + 1721), or expressed as an odds, it is 55:1721, which simplifies to 1:31 (called OAPR).

NB:
Disorder: cranial haematoma.
Prognostic marker: skull X-ray.
Marker (test) positive: skull fracture.
What happens to 'positives': further investigations, such as CT scan after hospital admission.

low incidence of haematoma in people who are not disoriented (only 0.05% or 1 in 2000).

In those who are disoriented, the association between the marker and disorder is more modest (odds ratio 35) but still represents a large effect. The DR increases to 77%, but the FPR is much larger (9% instead of 1%). Skull X-rays therefore appear initially as a less effective prognostic marker in these particular patients (LR=8.5), but the OAPR is 1:3 (357:1214 or absolute risk 22.7%). (Alternatively, 22.7% of disorientated people with a skull fracture have a haematoma.) This means that there would only be three unnecessary additional investigations in people without a haematoma in order to detect one affected case. Even though the marker (skull X-ray) seems to have a lower prognostic performance in these patients than those who are not disorientated, when applied to the population, it becomes worthwhile because of the higher background incidence (1 in 30, 461/13, 680)).

This example shows the importance of not only looking at prognostic performance (DR and FPR), but also how well the marker works in a population (OAPR, or absolute risk). The adjusted OR is important because it has allowed for potential confounding factors, so burn size seems to be an independent risk factor.

Example 9.2 Burn size and mortality
In this example, the prognostic marker is a continuous factor. The study was a prospective cohort based on admissions to a single hospital between January 1998 and September 2008 [12] of 952 children with burns covering at least 30% of their total body surface area (TBSA). Burn size (measured by TBSA) was the prognostic marker, and the outcome was mortality (123 died).

The OR for dying among patients with a burn size of ≥60% (compared with burn size <60%) is high: 10.07 (95% CI 5.56–19.22), after allowing for other factors (inhalation injury, gender, age at admission, and time from the burn injury to admission). The adjusted OR is best to use: burn size seems to be an independent risk factor.

Figure 9.2a shows how DR (sensitivity) and FPR (1 – specificity) change as the burn size cut-off increases from 30.25% up to almost 100%. Using markers of the type used in Example 9.1, in which the result can only take one of two levels (normal or abnormal), it is not possible to change the DR or FPR. However, with a continuous marker, such as burn size, it is possible to change prognostic performance. As the DR increases, so too does the FPR. A **receiver operating characteristic** (ROC) curve is commonly shown for this type of prognostic marker (Figure 9.2b), and a quantitative measure of performance is the **area under the curve** (AUC), also known as the **concordance index ('c')**. The AUC value is the chance that the marker will produce a higher risk value for an individual with the outcome than someone without the outcome. If the marker is useless, DR and FPR are the same, as indicated by the line of identity in Figure 9.2b; the AUC would be 0.5 (i.e. the area for the whole square plot is 1.0, and the line of identity represents half of this). The higher the AUC, the better the prognostic marker. In the example, the AUC is 0.81, which is acceptable.

Although AUC is commonly used, it is unit-less, and its clinical relevance is not obvious. DR and FPR are better measures to interpret, and these are shown in Table 9.3. The authors selected a burn size cut-off of ≥62%, which is where the curves for DR and FPR cross (Figure 9.2a). This is the statistically most efficient point, but in practice, the cut-off is chosen after agreeing a suitable DR, for which the FPR is then fixed, or vice versa. Hence, tables like Table 9.3 are very useful when examining prognostic markers. The choice of cut-off depends on how important it is to identify as many cases as possible but also what happens to false positives. If it is more important to have high DR, then having a high FPR might be acceptable. But if the additional tests or interventions among those who are marker positive are harmful or very expensive, it might be more important to keep the FPR low, accepting that the DR would not be high.

From Table 9.3, the DR is 74% for ~26% FPR using the cut-off of ≥62% (i.e. 74% of those who died had a burn size of ≥62%, while 26% of those who did not die have a burn size of this magnitude). The OAPR 1:2.3 (absolute risk or PPV of 30%). Referring three patients (who do not later die) immediately to a specialist unit for every one that dies seems worthwhile, particularly if the death can be prevented.

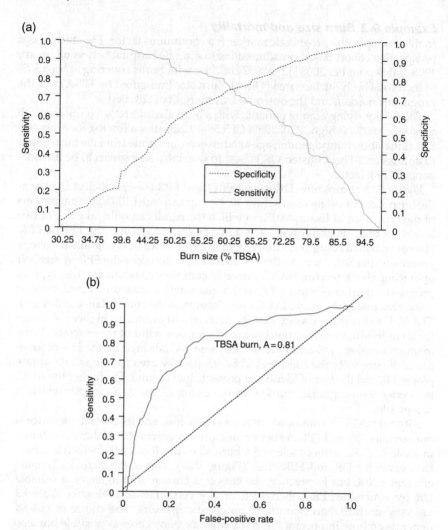

Figure 9.2 DR (sensitivity) and FPR (1 – specificity) in relation to burn size (% of TBSA). The lower diagram is a plot of DR against FPR, called an ROC curve, from which the AUC (A) is 0.81. Both diagrams can be used to develop Table 9.3. Source: Kraft et al., 2012 [12]. Reproduced by permission of Elsevier.

An important consideration is that all patients received the same maximum treatment in this single-centre study, so the relationship between burn size cut-off and the mortality rate might be different from that in other centres. Consequently, the OAPR may not be generalisable, because this depends on the background death rate: if this is higher elsewhere, then the OAPR becomes more favourable (or less favourable with a lower death rate).

Table 9.3 Prognostic performance for fixed FPR cut-offs using Figure 9.2.

FPR (%)	Approximate DR (%)	Approximate burn size cut-off (% TBSA)	Estimated OAPR (absolute risk %)
10	43	76	1:1.6 (38)
20	63	66	1:2.1 (32)
26	74	62	1:2.3 (30)
30	80	57	1:2.5 (29)
40	82	52	1:3.3 (23)
50	89	49	1:3.8 (21)

OAPR, odds of being affected given a positive result, using the 123 deaths and 829 who did not die (i.e. background risk is 123:829 or 1:6.7).
FPR is 10% (0.10), meaning that 10% of unaffected (alive) individuals are picked up (flagged), while 43% (DR, 0.43) of those who eventually die are identified.
The OAPR is $0.43 \times 1 : 6.7 \times 0.10$, which simplifies to 1:1.6.
To identify every child that dies, 1.6 children who do not die are (flagged) for specialist care.
OAPR of 1:1.6 is the same as an absolute risk of $1/(1 + 1.6) = 38\%$.

NB:
Disorder: mortality.
Prognostic marker: measuring burn size (as % of TBSA).
Marker (test) positive: burn size $\geq$ a specified cut-off (e.g. 60%).
What happens to 'positives': immediate referral to a specialised burn care unit, with close monitoring and effective treatments given.

Outcome measures based on 'taking measurements on people' (continuous endpoints)

Prognostic analyses generally aim to estimate the risk or chance of developing an outcome, but there is no concept of risk when dealing with a continuous measurement. For example, a body weight of 85 kg, or blood pressure value of 110 mmHg, is simply a measurement. They can, however, be converted into risk by categorising the factor. For example, body weight can be divided into two groups (<100 and $\geq$100 kg), and the risk associated with having a large weight considered. The same approaches can then be used as in the previous section (page 177). Alternatively, a linear regression could be used[#] with the outcome measure in its original form, but this only measures association and the ability to predict values of the continuous outcome for individuals and does not provide risk results. Also, the concepts of OR and FPR do not readily apply, because there are no defined separate groups of affected and unaffected individuals.

Outcome measures based on time-to-event data

If the outcome measure is a time-to-event factor, it is simplest to specify a time point (e.g. 1 year), so that anyone who has had the event by 1 year is classified as 'affected' and anyone who has not is classified as 'unaffected'. Dividing the outcome data into these two groups allows the same approach to be used as in the previous section (page 177). However, to do this, all study participants

---

[#]Or multivariable regression, when considering several factors together used for prediction.

must have been followed up by at least 1 year, unless they have had the event (outcome) of interest before.

Example 9.3 Smooth muscle actin and survival

This example is based on a translational study using clinical data extracted from patient records and stored tissue (cancer) samples, that is, a retrospective study [13]. All patients had oral cancer and had had surgical treatment to remove the tumour. There were 282 consecutively selected patients (1992–2005) who had complete data on survival and several key potential prognostic factors and for whom the archival pathology sample was available. The prognostic marker of interest is a biomarker called smooth muscle actin (SMA, measured in the tumour sample), the previous section (page X) low, medium, or high expression. Classification into the three categories was performed *centrally, independently* by two histopathologists, using *standardised criteria*, important design features of biomarker studies, particularly if it is a new marker. The measurement is semi-quantitative, in that the histopathologist estimates the percentage of 'stromal positivity' in each tissue sample (<5, 5–50, and >50% for the three groups, respectively). As this is only an approximation, the categorisation was considered necessary to avoid having a continuous marker that appears to be measured precisely, when this is not the case. Usually continuous factors should be kept as they are in the analysis. The outcome measure here is time until death from oral cancer. There were 120 deaths.

Figure 9.3 presents the Kaplan–Meier curves for SMA and death. Such diagrams are useful because they illustrate the association, in this case a clear

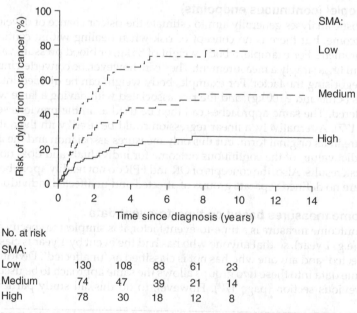

No. at risk					
SMA:					
Low	130	108	83	61	23
Medium	74	47	39	21	14
High	78	30	18	12	8

Figure 9.3 Kaplan–Meier curves for the association between a tumour prognostic marker SMA and death from oral cancer, among oral cancer patients.

Table 9.4 Prognostic performance for SMA and its ability to predict death from oral cancer at either 1 or 3 years.

SMA group	1-year status			3-year status		
	DR (%)	FPR (%)	LR	DR (%)	FPR (%)	LR
	60 deaths	214 alive		99 deaths	164 alive	
Medium or high	73	47	1.6	73	40	1.8
High only	47	22	2.1	47	13	3.6

DR, detection rate; FPR, false-positive rate; LR, likelihood ratio (DR/FPR).

NB:
Disorder: death from oral cancer, among patients diagnosed with this disorder.
Prognostic marker: measuring SMA in the removed tumour sample.
Marker (test) positive: SMA medium or high.
What happens to 'positives': further investigations, closer monitoring, or treatments to reduce the chance of dying.

trend from low to high SMA. Compared with low SMA, the unadjusted hazard ratio for medium SMA is 2.18 (95% CI 1.35–3.51); for high SMA, it is 4.26 (95% CI 2.74–6.61).

To examine DR and FPR, the 1-year survival time point was specified, producing two groups: dead by 1 year and alive at 1 year (similarly at 3 years). A death after this time point would not be counted as an event. Only patients who had died before 1 year (n=60) or those who had been followed up for at least 1 year (n=214) could be included. Having to exclude individuals because they have not had enough follow-up is a problem with retrospective analyses. Table 9.4 shows the prognostic performance for SMA on its own. Although the measures of association using hazard ratios are reasonable (2.18 and 4.26), the DR and FPR are not satisfactory: either the DR is high (73%) but with high FPR (47%), or the DR is moderate (47%) but with lower FPR (22%). The LRs are too small to make SMA alone a worthwhile marker.

There are several other known prognostic markers for mortality among these patients (such as disease stage, and whether or not the cancer has metastasised), so these need to be allowed for. Because SMA on its own is not a good prognostic marker, the next step is to consider it with these other markers to produce a prognostic model (next section).

9.5 Examining several factors to develop a prognostic model

There are many situations where several markers are investigated, and the 'best' subset of these is used to develop a model for predicting outcomes (with multivariable logistic or Cox regression analyses).

The following steps can be performed:
• Examine effect sizes, such as odds or hazards ratio, in all study participants to acquire an understanding of the markers (a measure of association with the outcome).

Table 9.5 Hazard ratios for selected markers from Example 9.3 (oral cancer patients).

	Unadjusted hazard ratio (95% CI)	Adjusted hazard ratio (95% CI)[#]	p-value (from multivariable Cox regression)
Age			
For increase of 5 yrs	1.04 (0.97–1.11)	1.08 (0.99–1.16)	0.07
Disease stage			
I	1.0	1.0	0.20
II	2.61 (1.41–4.82)	1.90 (0.99–3.66)	
III	3.02 (1.34–6.82)	1.62 (0.65–4.03)	
IV	3.64 (2.24–5.94)	1.21 (0.62–2.33)	
Metastases			
No	1.0	1.0	0.05
Yes	2.31 (1.61–3.32)	1.76 (1.00–3.11)	
Pattern of invasion			
Cohesive	1.0	1.0	0.001
Discohesive	2.46 (1.71–3.54)	2.07 (1.33–3.24)	
Depth of invasion			
For increase of 5 yrs	1.40 (1.23–1.59)	0.96 (0.78–1.19)	0.71
SMA expression			
Low	1.0	1.0	0.002
Medium	2.18 (1.35–3.51)	2.01 (1.14–3.52)	
High	4.26 (2.74–6.61)	3.06 (1.65–5.66)	

[#] Altogether there were 15 markers in the full analyses (all used in the multivariable model that produced the adjusted hazard ratios) [13].

- Develop the model in a training dataset.
- Test the model in a separate validation dataset, that is, obtain estimates of prognostic performance.
- Validate the model, that is, check that the model is reliable.

The first three of these stages are illustrated using Example 9.3 [13]. Altogether, 15 markers (some of which were already known to be associated with survival) were analysed. Table 9.5 shows the hazard ratios for selected markers for illustrative purposes. For example, depth of invasion on its own, has a statistically significant association with survival (hazard ratio 1.40), but not when adjusted for other markers (0.96). The hazard ratios for disease stage reduce and become non-statistically significant, though they still appear raised (the lack of significance could be due to insufficient sample size). There is some evidence for an association with metastases and pattern of invasion, possibly with age, but no clear trend for disease stage.

The adjusted hazard ratios were 2.01 and 3.06, for medium and high SMA, respectively. They are lower than the unadjusted values, but still show a reasonably good association with mortality.

The next step is to determine which subset, of all 15 markers, best predicts survival. Manually selecting only those markers that are statistically significant from Table 9.5 will not necessarily yield the best model, so this approach should be avoided. Markers that seem ineffective individually, may actually be useful when combined with others. Before the model is developed, the dataset is divided into two groups: training and validation. In Example 9.3, the division was based on time, so the first two-thirds of events were in the training set (patients diagnosed up to and including 9 October 2002) and the last third in the validation set (after 9 October 2002). This produced a sufficient number of oral cancer deaths in each group: 80 (among 163 patients) and 40 (among 116 patients), that is, a 2:1 ratio for the number of events.[#]

Another Cox regression is then performed in the training dataset using all 15 markers to identify a subset that might together produce a good prognostic model [14]. The selection is done within the regression analyses using a method called **backward elimination**, with a threshold level of statistical significance of 5% (10% could be used instead, if researchers wish to be more permissive and potentially include more factors in the final model). There are two other methods of selecting a subset of variables, stepwise or forward selection, but backward elimination is generally preferred because it can yield a combination of markers that have a better performance. Beginning with all 15 markers, each is omitted in turn, and the marker that has the least impact on the model (assessed using a statistical criterion) is excluded. This analysis is repeated using the remaining 14 markers, and again, the aim is to drop one marker. The process continues until removing a factor has an impact (i.e. the change in model adequacy becomes statistically significant at the 5 or 10% level). This then forms the final model. This entire process is performed automatically within the analysis. In the example, the backward elimination analysis produced four markers, shown in Table 9.6 with their regression coefficients (i.e. the $\log_e$ hazard ratios). At this stage, it is worth checking that the effect sizes in the training dataset are similar to those based on the whole dataset (Table 9.5). For models using logistic regression, the coefficients would be $\log_e$ odds ratios.

Age was not statistically significant in Table 9.5 (in either the unadjusted or adjusted estimates), but was selected in the final model. This confirms that factors should not be manually selected based on individual p-values. In the selection process, the factors are chosen for the model on purely statistical grounds. The researchers may feel that some excluded markers are clinically important, in which case they could be added back to the model.

A check of the adequacy of the final model could be done (see page 79).

The coefficients in Table 9.6 are then used as 'scores' to be applied to patients in the validation dataset (see table footnote). The score is, essentially, a single variable, for which cut-off points can be selected to examine DR and FPR, in a similar way as burn size was analysed in Example 9.2. For outcome measures that are time-to-event factors, a fixed time point should be specified (here 3-year mortality). There are statistical methods to estimate DR and FPR using censored time-to-event data [15, 16].

[#] There were missing data for 3 of the original total of 282 patients.

Table 9.6 Results of a backward elimination analysis (Cox regression) of 15 potential prognostic markers for mortality among oral cancer patients.

Marker	Regression coefficient*	Odds ratio (exponential of the coefficient)
SMA expression		
Low	0	1.0
Medium	0.731	2.08
High	1.186	3.27
Age (for increase of 1 year)	0.0226	1.02
Metastatic disease status		
No metastases	0	1.0
With metastases	0.585	1.79
Tumour cohesion		
Cohesive	0	1.0
Discohesive	0.899	2.46

Reference category has coefficient of 0 (hazard ratio of 1.0).
*These become scores to estimate prognostic performance using the patients in the validation dataset (i.e. the regression model is used to predict a combined score based on all four markers).

Examples of calculating a score:
Patient 1 has medium SMA, an age of 65, no metastases, and discohesive tumour invasion.
Patient 2 has high SMA, an aged of 73, metastases, and discohesive tumour invasion.
Patient 3 has low SMA, an age of 69, no metastases, and cohesive tumour invasion.

	SMA	Age	Metastases	Cohesion	Total score
Patient 1	0.731+	0.0226×65+	0+	0.899	3.10
Patient 2	1.186+	0.0226×73+	0.585+	0.899	4.32
Patient 3	0+	0.0226×69+	0+	0	1.56

Higher total scores would be associated with higher risk of dying.

In Example 9.3, there were 116 patients (40 oral cancer deaths) in the validation dataset. Figure 9.4 is the ROC curve based on the four markers in Table 9.6. As in Example 9.2, a table of DRs and FPRs could be derived from the figure, so that researchers can select the one they consider to have the best balance. For DR of 70%, the corresponding FPR is 20%:

- 70% of those who died by 3 years were classified as marker (test) positive.
- 20% of those who did not die by 3 years were classified as marker (test) positive.

This performance is clearly better than SMA on its own or indeed any other established prognostic marker individually. Although these findings suggest that there could be an effective model using the four factors, the study was retrospective, so they should be examined prospectively before any firm conclusions can be made.

The next important step is to validate the model by comparing observed with expected risks. This is best done using a completely new dataset from the one used to develop the model and examine initial estimates of performance.

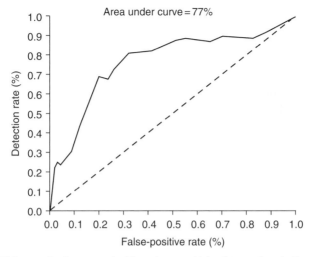

Figure 9.4 ROC curve (for 3 year survival) based on combining four markers in Example 9.3.

Example 9.4 Maternal serum markers and Down's Syndrome

Figure 9.5 shows an example validating risk using antenatal screening for Down's syndrome. The prognostic model was based on maternal age and measurement of four serum markers in maternal blood, which, together, were combined into a risk score (i.e. a single continuous factor, similar to that in Example 9.2). The serum markers were measured in stored samples (from a biobank), which came from a case–control study of 75 Down's syndrome and 367 unaffected pregnancies, matched for maternal age, gestational age, and duration of storage of the serum sample, plus samples from 970 Caucasian women with unaffected pregnancies [9]. The model was developed on this dataset, and later validated in a completely independent dataset of 19,597 women of whom 47 had a confirmed Down's syndrome pregnancy [17]. The risk score is divided into five groups, and the mean predicted risk from the model is calculated in each group. This is compared with the observed prevalence of affected births in each group. There is an excellent agreement between the two, confirming that the prognostic model is valid. Such analyses are often only reliable when the validation study is suitably large, and in particular has a sufficient number of events.

9.6 Genetic studies

Genetic studies are often used to examine prognostic markers that are genes, a genetic mutation or a DNA variant, such as a single-nucleotide polymorphism (SNP), which may or may not be directly causally related to a disorder or poor outcome, but is assumed to be associated with a gene that is related.

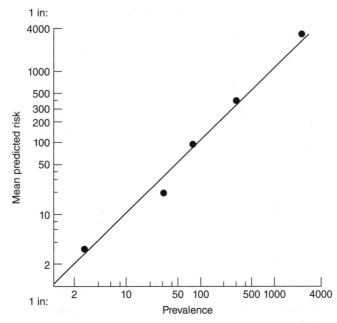

Figure 9.5 Validating a prognostic model: comparison of the mean predicted risk based on a model of five factors, when applied to a completely new dataset of 19,597 pregnancies, which included 47 with Down's syndrome. The diagonal line represents perfect agreement between observed and expected prevalence. Source: Wald et al., 1996 [17]. Reproduced by permission of SAGE publishers (Copyright Allan Hackshaw).

Two types of studies have been conducted:
1. Family-based studies, based on examining and comparing genetic loci among related individuals, often first-degree relatives
2. Population-based studies of large numbers of individuals, to examine the relationship between genetic markers and a disorder

The basic study designs are essentially the same as those presented in Chapters 5–7, and in many cases, the genetic work is a subsidiary analysis of an observational study that was conducted for a different purpose. A summary of issues specific to genetic studies is given in a series in *The Lancet* [18–24] and elsewhere [25–28]. Box 9.2 shows some key considerations (see also Box 1.12).

The simplest type of analysis is to examine the association between the presence or absence of a genetic mutation (e.g. BRCA1) and a disorder (e.g. whether or not a woman develops breast cancer). This can be done using a 2 × 2 table, from which an odds ratio and 95% CI can be calculated and interpreted, as in Table 6.2.

Box 9.2 Some key considerations for studies examining genetic factors (markers)

• Appropriate informed consent must be obtained from study participants (see Chapter 11, page 220).
• Data confidentiality must be ensured.
• The consequences for study participants (i.e. whether or not genetic results could or would be reported back to them) must be specified.
• Specify where the study participants come from, and that they represent the target population of interest.
• There must be reliable measurement of genetic markers (using validated techniques and equipment).
• Quantification and assessment of the genotyping call rate (the percentage of all genotypes that give non-missing values) should be in place.
• There must be good quality control of the genotyping processes in the laboratory.
• Screening of many thousands of SNPs can produce several false positives (i.e. an SNP considered to be associated with a disorder but in reality it is not), so it is important that the selected SNPs are subsequently examined in an independent dataset.
• The effect size between an SNP and a disorder is usually moderate or small (odds or hazard ratio <1.30), so to find a statistically significant result at very small levels (e.g. $p < 0.00001$), large studies are required.

Linkage studies

The purpose of several genetic studies is to find a DNA marker (e.g. an SNP) that is always present (carried) in those family members with the disorder and absent in those who are unaffected. When this is achieved, the marker and the gene likely to cause the disorder are said to be linked, and they probably lie close together on the chromosome. Researchers then try to find the actual gene, or gene variant, of interest in subsequent studies.

Linkage studies are usually based on large families, which include people with and without the disorder of interest and, ideally, where the disease has affected people over several generations. Extending the study beyond first-degree relatives can be useful, but is sometimes difficult in practice, because a DNA sample must be obtained from all study participants. Such studies may require significant resources to track down relatives and obtain blood samples and other information (e.g. demographics) on them.

Specialist computing software is used to analyse linkage studies (with modelling such as maximum likelihood or non-parametric methods).

Genome-wide association studies

Linkage studies examine the relationship between a genetic marker and a gene (gene variant) that is likely to cause a disorder. Genome-wide association (GWA) studies try to locate the gene by examining the relationship between the disorder and the gene markers. The markers are scanned across the complete set of DNA, or genomes, for each study individual (hence the term **genome-wide**). All of the study designs described in this book have been used for this, though the best design is a prospective cohort, because it can measure risk, collect sufficient data on the study participants (minimising missing data), and attempt to obtain a sample for DNA analysis on all. Many GWA studies are based on unrelated participants, but some include family-based groups. With improved and cheaper technology, the scope for measuring genome-wide markers has grown, and GWA studies are becoming more common.

An important consideration is that the study participants are representative of the target population to minimise or avoid selection bias. Also, case–control studies need to ensure adequate matching for ethnic background or only focus on a relatively homogenous ethnic group.

GWA studies usually involve measuring several thousand SNPs, each a potential prognostic marker, so the interpretation of such studies is different from those described in Chapters 5–7, in which the focus was on a single or a few well-defined exposures. Multiple testing and finding associations that are due to chance are important considerations in conducting GWA analyses. When interpreting the selected SNPs, a statistical significance level of $p = 0.05$ is too large to make conclusions, so only SNPs that have very small p-values are considered to have a real association. One of the main issues is finding false positives: SNPs that appear to have an association with a disorder, when in reality they do not. This can be addressed by ensuring that SNPs are evaluated in an independent dataset to confirm both the presence of the association and the size of the effect.

Table 9.7 is an example of a case control study examining a single SNP (labelled as rs2476601, C1858T) and its relationship with rheumatoid arthritis, [29]. This SNP lies close to the PTPN22 gene, which provides coding for the PTPN22 protein, associated with immune response. The allele of interest is T (i.e. this is thought to increase the risk of the disorder). Before analysing the data, the Hardy–Weinberg Equilibrium (HWE) should be checked, particularly in the control group. If HWE does not hold, this may indicate systematic genotyping errors or other biases, and so the study findings could be

Table 9.7 Association between a single SNP variant and a disorder (rheumatoid arthritis): Controls were healthy individuals without rheumatoid arthritis [29].

	Number with genotype (%)			Frequency of the T allele* (%)
	CC	CT	TT	
Cases (n = 302)	218 (72.2)	72 (23.8)	12 (0.4)	15.9
Controls (n = 374)	312 (83.4)	61 (16.3)	1 (0.3)	8.4
Odds ratio (95% CI)	1.0	1.69 (1.15–2.48)	17.17 (2.49–736)**	

*(0.5 × CT percentage) + TT percentage.
**Estimated using Fisher's exact test because of small numbers.

questionable. In the example, a test for observed versus expected frequencies, assuming HWE, yields p-values of 0.06 and 0.267 for cases and controls, respectively (both >0.05) [26], though the one for controls is perhaps more important because these do not have the disorder and so they should represent the general population.

The table shows that the frequency of the T allele is greater among cases than controls. A chi-squared test for the association yields $p < 0.001$, and a test for trend from CC to TT could also be performed ($p < 0.001$). These observations suggest that there is a reasonably strong statistical relationship between this SNP and the risk of rheumatoid arthritis.

In GWA studies, each SNP, out of many thousand, is analysed separately. The selected SNPs could then be analysed using multivariable logistic regression, in which the outcome measure is the presence or absence of the disorder of interest, and each SNP is included in the model as a separate factor. The model then produces an odds ratio for each SNP, allowing for the effects of all the others. Selection methods (e.g. backward elimination or stepwise selection) could be used to find a subset of markers, which, together, produce a good model. An alternative approach is to combine data on each SNP from several studies using meta-analytical techniques (Chapter 10), but this does not involve examination of two or more SNPs simultaneously. More advanced statistical methods could be used to analyse the relationship between a disorder that is caused by several gene variants and statistical interactions between genes.

For most SNPs and disorders, the effect size is expected to be moderate, or small (odds or hazard ratios <1.30). Therefore, large studies are required to examine these associations reliably and to allow for multiple (several thousand) comparisons. Sample size calculations can be performed using the expected allele frequency and assuming modest odds (or hazards) ratios (e.g. see Figure 7.3). Consequently, GWA studies are usually a collaboration among several research teams, who have each conducted a study separately and who then pool their data and biological samples.

Figure 9.6 shows an example of a large GWA study, which aimed to find genes associated with the risk of developing multiple sclerosis [30]. There were 334,923 SNPs initially analysed, and to address this, the researchers created two separate datasets: a screening set, to find a subset of SNPs that seem to have a relationship with risk (quantified using odds ratios), and another, to replicate the findings (i.e. to confirm whether or not similar odds ratios and statistical significance are found). The final set of SNPs was then analysed using the combined screening and replication datasets, because this should produce the most reliable effect sizes and smallest p-values (Table 9.8). Unlike examples covered in Chapters 5–7, in which there is a pre-defined exposure, and so the p-value often just needs to be <0.05, conclusions on SNPs are only made using the smallest p-values, for example, $3.0 \times 10^{-8\#}$ for the SNP rs12722489 (and gene IL2RA). The table shows the type of information required for a typical GWA study, and in this example, the results for four

---

0.00000003.

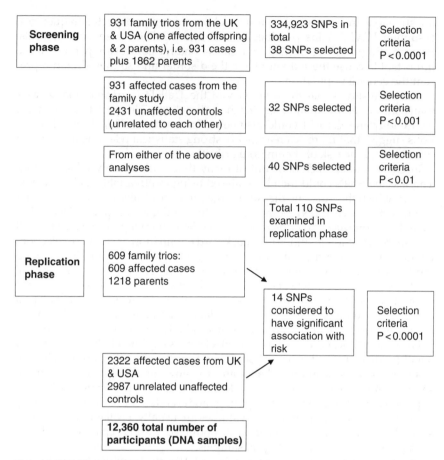

Figure 9.6 Outline of a GWA study of multiple sclerosis, which aimed to find SNPs with strong associations with the risk of multiple sclerosis. Data from Ref. [30].

SNPs and three genes. It is noted that in the screening phase analyses effect sizes were produced separately for related and unrelated study individuals. The odds ratios do not indicate strong associations, with the largest one being only 1.25, indicating that individuals with the 'C' allele for the SNP rs12722489 (associated with the gene IL2RA) have a 25% increased risk of having multiple sclerosis.

9.7 Key points

• A prognostic marker can be any clinical or personal characteristic, a biomarker or genetic marker in biological samples, or an imaging test.
• Evaluating an exposure as a prognostic marker requires several statistical considerations: measure of association and prognostic performance.

Table 9.8 Selected SNPs (and genes), found to have an association with the risk of multiple sclerosis [31].

Gene	SNP	Risk allele	Frequency of allele (%)	Screening phase				Replication phase		All study participants (n = 12,360)	
				Family trios		Cases from family trios plus unrelated controls		Another set of family trios and unrelated controls			
				Odds ratio (95% CI)	p-value	Odds ratio (95% CI)	p-value	Odds ratio (95% CI)	p-value	Odds ratio (95% CI)	p-value
IL2RA	rs12722489	C	85	1.35 (1.13–1.62)	1.3×10^{-3}	1.30 (1.11–1.52)	9.6×10^{-4}	1.19 (1.08–1.31)	4.6×10^{-4}	1.25 (1.16–1.36)	3.0×10^{-8}
IL2RA	rs2104286	T	75	1.26 (1.08–1.47)	3.2×10^{-3}	1.26 (1.11–1.43)	2.8×10^{-4}	1.16 (1.08–1.25)	1.5×10^{-4}	1.19 (1.11–1.26)	2.2×10^{-7}
IL7R	rs6897932	C	75	1.24 (1.07–1.44)	5.8×10^{-3}	1.17 (1.03–1.32)	1.6×10^{-2}	1.18 (1.09–1.27)	2.7×10^{-5}	1.18 (1.11–1.26)	2.9×10^{-7}
KIAA0350	rs6498169	G	37	1.16 (1.02–1.33)	2.9×10^{-2}	1.17 (1.04–1.31)	6.5×10^{-3}	1.16 (1.09–1.24)	1.9×10^{-5}	1.14 (1.08–1.21)	3.8×10^{-6}

Key observations:
- SNPs identified as having an association with multiple sclerosis in the screening phase were confirmed using the replication dataset (the odds ratios were still raised and highly statistically significant).
- For two SNPs (first two rows of the table), the size of the association is smaller in the replication dataset.
- The final analysis (based on all participants) provides the most reliable estimates of odds ratio, again smaller for the two SNPs.

- Measures of association are relative risk, odds ratio, and hazard ratio (all interpreted in the same way as in other chapters); measures of prognostic performance are DR (sensitivity), FPR (1 – specificity), and OAPR (or PPV).
- When considering several potential markers, they must be combined using a model (usually logistic or Cox regression).
- These models need to be derived and tested on separate datasets, and a check needs to be made that estimated (predicted) and observed risk values are similar.
- Using a single continuous marker or a model based on several markers, DR and FPR will both increase or decrease together.
- Choosing an appropriate DR and FPR depends on several factors, including the importance (severity) of the disorder and what happens to marker positives (particularly false positives).
- Studies of genetic markers have similar designs to other types of exposures, but the interpretation of results is different because of multiple testing (when several hundred or thousand SNPs are examined).

References

1. Moons KG, Royston P, Vergouwe Y, Grobbee DE, Altman DG. Prognosis and prognostic research: what, why, and how? BMJ 2009;338:b375.
2. Royston P, Moons KG, Altman DG, Vergouwe Y. Prognosis and prognostic research: developing a prognostic model. BMJ 2009;338:b604.
3. Altman DG, Vergouwe Y, Royston P, Moons KG. Prognosis and prognostic research: validating a prognostic model. BMJ 2009;338:b605.
4. Moons KG, Altman DG, Vergouwe Y, Royston P. Prognosis and prognostic research: application and impact of prognostic models in clinical practice. BMJ 2009;338:b606.
5. Moons KG, Kengne AP, Woodward M, Royston P, Vergouwe Y, Altman DG, Grobbee DE. Risk prediction models: I. Development, internal validation, and assessing the incremental value of a new (bio) marker. Heart 2012;98(9):683–90.
6. Moons KG, Kengne AP, Grobbee DE, Royston P, Vergouwe Y, Altman DG, Woodward M. Risk prediction models: II. External validation, model updating, and impact assessment. Heart 2012;98(9):691–8.
7. Vergouwe Y, Royston P, Moons KG, Altman DG. Development and validation of a prediction model with missing predictor data: a practical approach. J Clin Epidemiol 2010;63(2):205–14.
8. Wald NJ, Hackshaw AK, Frost C. When can a risk factor be used as a worthwhile screening test? BMJ 1999;319:1562–5.
9. Wald NJ, Densem JW, Smith D, Klee GG. Four-marker serum screening for Down's syndrome. Prenat Diagn 1994;14(8):707–16.
10. Peduzzi P, Concato J, Kemper E, Holford TR, Feinstein AR. A simulation study of the number of events per variable in logistic regression analysis. J Clin Epidemiol 1996; 49(12):1373–9.
11. Mendelow AD, Teasdale G, Jennett B, Bryden J, Hessett C, Murray G. Risks of intracranial haematoma in head injured adults. Br Med J (Clin Res Ed) 1983;287(6400):1173–6.
12. Kraft R, Herndon DN, Al-Mousawi AM, Williams FN, Finnerty CC, Jeschke MG. Burn size and survival probability in paediatric patients in modern burn care: a prospective observational cohort study. Lancet 2012;379(9820):1013–21.
13. Marsh D, Suchak K, Moutasim KA, Vallath S, Hopper C, Jerjes W, et al. Stromal activation predicts for clinically aggressive oral cancer. J Pathol 2011;223(4):470–81.

14. Greenland S. Modeling and variable selection in epidemiologic analysis. Am J Public Health 1989;79(3):340–9.

15. Lu L, Liu C. Using the time dependent ROC curve to build a better survival model in SAS. North East SAS Users group (NESUG), 2006; http://www.nesug.org/Proceedings/nesug06/an/da29.pdf. Accessed 20 May 2014.

16. Heagerty PJ, Lumley T, Pepe MS. Time dependent ROC curves for censored survival data and a diagnostic marker. Biometrics 2000;56:337–44.

17. Wald NJ, Hackshaw AK, Huttly W, Kennard A. Empirical validation of risk screening for Down's syndrome. J Medical Screen 1996;3(4):185–7.

18. Burton PR, Tobin MD, Hopper JL. Genetic epidemiology 1: key concepts in genetic epidemiology. Lancet 2005;366(9489):941–51. Erratum in: Lancet. 2006 Jan 7;367(9504):28.

19. Dawn TM, Barrett JH. Genetic epidemiology 2: genetic linkage studies. Lancet 2005;366(9490):1036–44.

20. Cordell HJ, Clayton DG. Genetic epidemiology 3: genetic association studies. Lancet 2005;366(9491):1121–31.

21. Palmer LJ, Cardon LR. Genetic epidemiology 4: shaking the tree: mapping complex disease genes with linkage disequilibrium. Lancet 2005;366(9492):1223–34.

22. Hattersley AT, McCarthy MI. Genetic epidemiology 5: what makes a good genetic association study? Lancet 2005;366(9493):1315–23.

23. Hopper JL, Bishop DT, Easton DF. Genetic epidemiology 6: population-based family studies in genetic epidemiology. Lancet 2005;366(9494):1397–406.

24. Davey SG, Ebrahim S, Lewis S, Hansell AL, Palmer LJ, Burton PR. Genetic epidemiology 7: genetic epidemiology and public health: hope, hype, and future prospects. Lancet 2005;366(9495):1484–98.

25. Lewis CM, Knight J. Introduction to genetic association studies. Cold Spring Harb Protoc 2012;2012(3):297–306. doi: 10.1101/pdb.top068163.

26. Amos CI. Successful design and conduct of genome-wide association studies. Hum Mol Genet. 2007;16(2):R220–5.

27. Rothman N, Hainaut P, Schulte P, Smith M, Boffetta P, Perera F. *Molecular Epidemiology: Principles and Practices.* International Agency for Research on Cancer (IARC) (2011).

28. McCarthy MI, Abecasis GR, Cardon LR, Goldstein DB, Little J, Ioannidis JP, Hirschhorn JN. Genome-wide association studies for complex traits: consensus, uncertainty and challenges. Nat Rev Genet 2008;9(5):356–69.

29. Steer S, Lad B, Grumley JA, Kingsley GH, Fisher SA. Association of R602W in a protein tyrosine phosphatase gene with a high risk of rheumatoid arthritis in a British population: evidence for an early onset/disease severity effect. Arthritis Rheum 2005;52(1):358–60.

30. Hafler DA, Compston A, Sawcer S, Lander ES, Daly MJ, De Jager PL, et al.; International Multiple Sclerosis Genetics Consortium. Risk alleles for multiple sclerosis identified by a genome wide study. N Engl J Med. 2007;357(9):851–62.

CHAPTER 10

Systematic reviews and meta-analyses

Chapters 5–8 provide an overview of the design and analysis of individual observational studies. Systematic reviews combine results from several published or unpublished studies, and are generally considered to provide more reliable evidence of an association than an individual study. Further reading on systematic reviews can be found elsewhere [1–6].

10.1 Dealing with inconsistent study findings

No two observational studies are identical in design and conduct, even if they have the same primary research objective. No single study should be used to change public health or clinical practice unless sufficiently large and conclusive. Ideally, there should be supporting evidence from two or more independent studies, in which the results are consistent. There are many occasions when results from different studies conflict, and the reasons must be investigated.

An example of inconsistent study results is illustrated in Table 10.1, which shows the key features and results from three observational studies examining the association between exposure to environmental tobacco smoke (passive smoking) among female never-smokers and the risk of lung cancer. The approach used here can be applied generally, that is, attempting to identify sources of bias and confounding, issues over study design and conduct, and biological plausibility.

The results cover all possible outcomes; one shows a clear positive association (i.e. exposure is associated with increased risk) [7], another suggests a protective effect (exposure associated with decreased risk) [8], and the third shows no evidence of an association in either direction [9]. Such discordant results may seem easily possible if the studies involved are small, but in this instance all three were relatively large (i.e. many participants and/or many cases of lung cancer).

The results from the Japanese study were as expected [7]. One key feature of causality is biological plausibility (see Box 2.6). The causal link between active smoking and lung cancer is well established, and exposure to environmental tobacco smoke involves breathing in the same carcinogenic substances as

A Concise Guide to Observational Studies in Healthcare, First Edition. Allan Hackshaw.

Table 10.1 Key design features and the main result from three observational studies of the association between passive smoking and the risk of lung cancer among female never-smokers.

Reference number	Design	Location	Recruitment period	No. of years' follow-up	No. with lung cancer	No. without lung cancer	Factors adjusted for	odds ratio (95% CI)*
7	Cohort	Japan	1965	16	200	91,340	Age	1.45 (1.02–2.08)
8	Case-control	China	1985–1987	Not applicable	417	602	Age, education, study area	0.7 (0.6–0.9)
9	Cohort	US	1959	39	177	25,765	Age, race, education, exercise, body mass index, urbanisation, fruit intake, health status	0.94 (0.66–1.33)

* Exposed to passive smoke versus unexposed.

active smoking. Another key feature is dose–response; smoking 20 cigarettes per day will have a higher risk than smoking 10, which in turn has a higher risk than smoking 5, and so on. Because it is generally accepted that there is no low level of exposure at which there is no excess risk of cancer, even smoking a single cigarette each day should be associated with some increased risk, compared with never-smokers, and evidence suggests that passive smoking could be equivalent to smoking about half a cigarette per day [10]. Therefore, there are robust scientific reasons for the association observed in the Japanese study.

The study from China [8] indicated that exposure to passive smoke *reduced* the risk of lung cancer by 30%, an odds ratio (OR) of 0.70 (Table 10.1). The 95% confidence interval (CI) excludes the no effect value 1.0, and the p-value, which was not reported in the publication, is estimated to be 0.005 or 0.02 if the upper limit was 0.94 rounded to 0.9 (using Box 6.8). Because this is statistically significant, it can be concluded that the effect was unlikely to be due to chance, if basing the interpretation on the p-value alone. However, no one would seriously claim that passive smoking could actually reduce the risk of lung cancer. In the study, heating and cooking practices increased lung cancer risk, which could have been exacerbated by a lack of ventilation (the women lived in northern China, which is very cold in winter). So it is possible that an association between passive smoking and lung cancer was blurred by other, more important risk factors. There is also the possibility that the effect was a chance finding in this particular study; a p-value of 0.005 means that an OR of 0.70 (or more extreme) could occur just by chance in 5 in 1000 studies of a similar size. This could, therefore, be one of those five studies. These hypotheses are, of course, unconfirmed.

The study from the US [9] requires more careful consideration. It was based on a subset of participants (in California), within a larger national cohort study, conducted in 25 US states. Initially, there seems to be nothing unusual about the study design or conduct, and in many situations, the large sample size (177 + 25,942) and long follow-up (39 years) would be considered as strengths. However, in this particular example, it is likely that after such a long follow-up, the exposure status has changed. Figure 10.1 shows how using only baseline exposure information could lead to a diluted effect. The exposure was whether women who were never-smokers did or did not live with a smoker, but this was ascertained at the start of the study (1959), and compared with the incidence of lung cancer over the subsequent 39 years. Because California had a high smoking quit rate, many women who were classified as 'exposed' at baseline were likely to have become unexposed later on (because their husbands quit smoking), and their risk of lung cancer should decrease to that of the original unexposed group. In the published results, 63% of ever smoking husbands were current smokers in 1959, compared with only 26% in 1998. A further consideration is that California had one of the highest divorce rates in the US, so women who were initially classified as exposed could have separated from their husband who smoked, and therefore no longer be exposed. These two features of the long follow-up could work

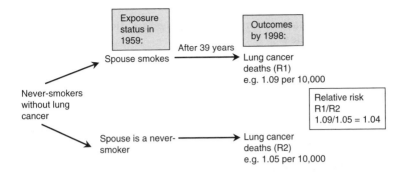

If exposure status had hardly changed over 39 years, R1 might have been1.37 per 10,000 (instead of 1.09). Then the relative risk of dying from lung cancer associated with having a spouse who smokes would be1.37/1.05:1.30 (i.e. a 30% increase in risk, consistent with many other similar studies).

However, if many couples had divorced after 1959, or many of the spouses who smoked in 1959 quit during the subsequent 39 years, the risk in the exposed group would get closer to that of the unexposed group (e.g. it could become 1.09 per 10,000), making the relative risk after such a long follow-up closer to 1.

Figure 10.1 Illustration of how changes in the exposure status could lead to an underestimated relative risk (using the study in Ref. [9]).

together to explain why there was no apparent increased risk associated with exposure to environmental tobacco smoke, in contrast to most other studies. However, it is also worth noting that the 95% CI was 0.66–1.33, so the upper limit allows for the possibility of an excess risk.

Interpreting and making conclusions about the results of a study can be relatively straightforward if they match the study hypotheses and are consistent with other studies and evidence. However, the example in Figure 10.1 shows that there are situations where this is not the case even when the study designs appear to be sufficiently reliable. It is important, to investigate such anomalies in study results, and attempt to find possible explanations. This can be done by further analyses of the data and by using evidence obtained elsewhere. Study results that seem to be inconsistent are a primary reason to perform a **systematic review**. In the case of the example such a review was conducted for 37 studies, which showed a clear and statistically significant excess risk of 24% (relative risk 1.24, 95% CI 1.13–1.36, p < 0.001) [11, 12]. This result was considered in the context of biological plausibility, other evidence, and with allowance for bias and confounding before concluding a causal association.

10.2 Systematic combination of studies

Large studies usually provide more robust results, allowing unambiguous conclusions to be made. In small studies, it can be difficult to detect an association, if one exists, and statistical significance is often not achieved (the

---

Box 10.1 Common reasons for performing systematic reviews of observational studies

To confirm existing practice but provide a more precise estimate of the association

By considering several studies together, the results are combined to give a single estimate of the effect size. The standard error (precision) of the pooled effect size is usually smaller than for any individual study, producing a narrow 95% CI and a result that is more likely to be statistically significant.

To change existing practice or public health education

A systematic review could lead to a new risk factor being included in public health education policies. Such reviews could be used to develop national guidelines for defining standard practice.

To determine whether new studies are needed

There might only be a few small published studies on a particular topic, and even a systematic review of them does not provide sufficient evidence; therefore, a large study is justified.

---

p-value is ≥ 0.05). This means that a real effect could be missed and there may be uncertainty over whether an observed result is real or due to chance.

The limitations of small studies could be largely overcome by combining them in a single analysis. This is one of the main purposes of a **systematic review**. Systematic reviews are different from review articles, which are often narratives, based on selected papers, and may therefore reflect the personal professional interests of the author. Review articles may incorporate a bias towards the positive (or negative) studies, and reviews tend to describe the features of each paper, without trying to combine the quantitative results. A valid assessment of several studies together needs to be conducted in a systematic and unbiased way.

Systematic reviews are generally considered to provide a better level of evidence than an individual study, and there are several reasons for undertaking them (Box 10.1).

10.3 What is a systematic review?

Systematic reviews are a formal methodological approach to obtaining, analysing, and interpreting all the available reports on a particular topic. In an era of evidence-based health, where health professionals are encouraged to identify sources of evidence for their work, and to keep abreast of new developments, systematic reviews are valuable summaries of the evidence. A review is only as good as the studies on which it is based. If an area has been

---

Box 10.2 Stages of a systematic review

1. Define the research question, and identify the appropriate outcome measures.
2. Specify a list of criteria for including and excluding studies.
3. Undertake a literature search (using medical databases, e.g. PubMed, Medline, and Embase), and identify articles that might be appropriate from the abstracts.
4. Obtain the full papers identified in the literature search. The reference lists of these papers could be used to identify additional papers not found in the electronic search.
5. Critically appraise each report and extract specific relevant information. Clearly defined outcome measures are essential.
6. Perform a **meta-analysis**, which involves combining the quantitative results from the individual studies into a single estimate.
7. Interpret and summarise the findings.

---

investigated mainly using small, poorly designed studies, a review of these may not be a substitute for a single large well-designed study.

A typical systematic review process is outlined in Box 10.2. The summary data (i.e. effect sizes) can be extracted from the published papers. Alternatively, the raw data might be requested from the authors; **Individual Patient Data (IPD) meta-analysis**. Data is sent to a central depository, essentially forming a single large dataset, with a variable that identifies each original study. One of the main advantages of IPD meta-analyses is that having the raw data allows subgroup analyses to be examined more reliably than using summary data from publications.

Systematic reviews can take from just a few weeks up to 2 or more years to complete, depending on how many studies there are and the type of meta-analysis to be conducted. Those based on IPD can be lengthy and require dedicated resources, because the raw data needs to be collected from each research group, collated, and checked before conducting the statistical analyses and writing the report.

10.4 Interpreting systematic reviews

Systematic reviews usually focus on studies that compare two or more groups of study participants, and can also be used to combine studies of a prognostic marker. The considerations when examining a review are:

- What is the aim of the review? This is often similar to the main objective of a single study.
- How was the review conducted?
- What are the main exposures and outcome measures?
- What are the main results?
- What are the implications for practice?

A first step is to summarise the key features of the studies in a table. This is illustrated in Table 10.2 using an example to be covered on page 209. Three important aspects are study design, study size, and which confounding factors were allowed for.

Figure 10.2 shows a typical meta-analysis plot (a **forest plot**), associated with a review of vitamin E and Parkinson's disease (Box 10.3) [14]. For plots like these, studies are usually listed in alphabetical order, according to the first author's surname, or by year of publication. However, it is more useful to order the studies by the magnitude of the effect size, making it easier to see how many studies lie below and above the no effect value, and the variation in effect sizes including possible outliers. Forest plots like the one shown in Figure 10.2 can be created using freely available software, RevMan [15].

Before the ORs are combined it is useful to see whether most or all of the studies lie in the same direction (i.e. above or below the no effect value). In Figure 10.2, five studies have an OR below 1.0 (moderate/high vitamin E intake is beneficial), and two have ORs above 1.0 (moderate/high vitamin E intake is harmful). Only one study (Zhang in Figure 10.2) had a statistically significant result on its own; all of the others did not. It is common to find variation in effect sizes and statistical significance, particularly when the study sizes vary considerably. Combining the studies, therefore, seems appropriate in order to produce a clearer conclusion about the association.

Meta-analysis

The main stage of a systematic review is combining the effect sizes into a single quantitative estimate using **meta-analysis** as the statistical technique. If a simple average of the effect sizes were taken, small and large studies would have the same influence in the analysis. There needs to be some way of taking into account, for example, that Zhang (2002) was based on $371 + 123,850$ participants and Scheider (1997) on only $57 + 50$ participants.

Large studies usually have small standard errors, which produce more precise estimates of the true effect size than those from studies with large standard errors. The **weight** given to each study is therefore calculated from the **standard error** of the OR or other effect size (Figure 10.3). In Figure 10.2, each weight is expressed as a percentage of the sum of all the weights across the seven studies, allowing a comparison of the relative contribution made by each study to the analysis. Forest plots usually make the size of the central square for the point estimate of each study proportional to the weight, so that studies with small standard errors have large squares making them more prominent.

Studies with small standard errors have narrow CIs and therefore large weights; in the example, Zhang (2002) with weight 28.4% (hence large square for the OR) is the largest study. Studies with large standard errors due to small sample size have the least weight, for example, Scheider (1997) (weight 4.1%, hence small square). Zhang (2002) will, therefore, have a greater influence in determining the combined OR than will Scheider (1997).

The size of the standard error, and the weight, depend on the number of events, as well as study size. For example, De Rijk (1997) has $31 + 5311$ participants but a slightly smaller weight (8.5%) than Anderson (1999) (11.3%),

Table 10.2 Studies examining the effect of maternal smoking on the risk of limb reduction defects (missing or deformed limbs, including missing, fused, or extra fingers or toes) [13].

First author	Study type	Source	Years	No. of unaffected infants	No. of cases	Unadjusted OR (95% CI)	Adjusted OR (95% CI)	Potential confounders	Matching variables for case-control studies
Aro (1983)	Case-control	Finnish Registry of Congenital Malformations	1964–1977	964,397*	453	1.4 (0.9–2.1)	1.30 (0.84–2.00)	M, A	B, L
Kricker (1986)	Case-control	Two Australian States	1970–1981	274	145	1.22 (0.76–1.96)	1.10 (0.64–1.90)	Pregnancy and maternal factors	B, L
Shiono (1986)	Cohort	Kaiser Permanente Birth Defects Study (US)	1974–1977	28,810	17	2.20 (0.83–5.80)	Stated as similar	M, R, A	
Van Den Eeden (1990)	Case-control	Washington State Birth Records (US)	1984–1986	4,323	35		1.20 (0.58–2.50)	M, P	B
Czeizel (1994)	Case-control	Hungarian Congenital Anomaly Register	1975–1984	537	537	2.02 (1.51–2.70)	1.68 (1.26–2.24)	E, P	B, L, G
Wasserman (1996)	Case-control	California Birth Defects Monitoring Program (US)	1987–1988	481	178	1.14 (0.77–1.69)	Stated as similar	R, P, A, MV	B, L
Kallen (2000)	Cohort	Swedish Registry of Congenital Malformations	1983–1996	1,387,192	1023	1.26 (1.10–1.44)	No adjustment		
Robitaille (2009)	Case-control	National Birth Defects Prevention Study (US)	1997–2003	4,956	527	1.11 (0.89–1.38)	No adjustment		

* Could have other defects.

Confounding or matching factors abbreviations:

M (maternal age), A (maternal alcohol use), R (race/ethnicity), P (parity or gravidity), E (maternal or paternal education), MV (periconceptional multivitamin supplementation including folic acid), B (birth month or year), L (location or study centre), G (infant gender).

NB: for Wasserman (1996), two factors were used to match controls to cases, but no factors were adjusted for in the statistical analysis.

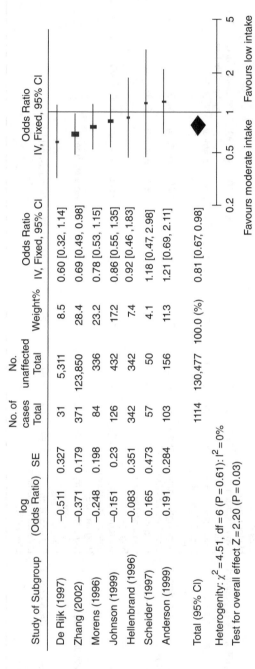

Study of Subgroup	log (Odds Ratio)	SE	No. of cases Total	No. unaffected Total	Weight%	Odds Ratio IV, Fixed, 95% CI	Odds Ratio IV, Fixed, 95% CI
De Rijk (1997)	−0.511	0.327	31	5,311	8.5	0.60 [0.32, 1.14]	
Zhang (2002)	−0.371	0.179	371	123,850	28.4	0.69 [0.49, 0.98]	
Morens (1996)	−0.248	0.198	84	336	23.2	0.78 [0.53, 1.15]	
Johnson (1999)	−0.151	0.23	126	432	17.2	0.86 [0.55, 1.35]	
Hellenbrand (1996)	−0.083	0.351	342	342	7.4	0.92 [0.46 ,1.83]	
Scheider (1997)	0.165	0.473	57	50	4.1	1.18 [0.47, 2.98]	
Anderson (1999)	0.191	0.284	103	156	11.3	1.21 [0.69, 2.11]	
Total (95% CI)			1114	130,477	100.0 (%)	0.81 [0.67, 0.98]	

Heterogenity: $\chi^2 = 4.51$, df = 6 (P = 0.61): $I^2 = 0\%$
Test for overall effect Z = 2.20 (P = 0.03)

Favours moderate intake   Favours low intake

Figure 10.2 Example of a forest plot from a meta-analysis: observational studies investigating the association between dietary vitamin E intake and Parkinson's disease (Box 10.3). The figure was obtained using RevMan. SE, standard error; cases, with Parkinson's disease; unaffected, without Parkinson's disease. Data from Ref. [14].

Box 10.3 Example of a systematic review [14]

Objective: To examine the association between dietary vitamin E and Parkinson's disease.

Design: Systematic review of observational studies published in 1996–2005, using a mixture of case–control (n = 5), cohort (n = 1), and cross-sectional studies (n = 1).

Eligibility: Studies were eligible for inclusion if there were a clear definition of vitamin E intake, clearly stated diagnostic criteria for Parkinson's disease, and potential confounders had been allowed for when estimating the OR (such as age, gender, and smoking).

Exposure: Dietary intake of vitamin E was based on the average reported daily intake of various food items and from vitamin supplements. Intake was defined according to quartiles or quintiles, and moderate/high intake was taken to be the second to fourth quartiles, or second to fifth quintiles. Comparison was then made with the lowest intake group.

Outcome measure: Presence or absence of Parkinson's disease.

Results: Figure 10.2.

Authors' conclusions: Vitamin E may have a neuroprotective effect on the risk of the disease, but the findings need confirmation in randomised controlled trials.

Weight is a measure of the relative importance of an individual study in a meta-analysis

Weight = 1/standard error^2

where the standard error is for any effect size, such as odds ratio, relative risk, hazard ratio, risk difference, or difference between two means

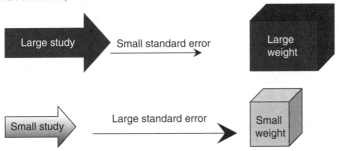

Figure 10.3 'Weight' of a study in a meta-analysis.

which has far fewer participants (103 + 156). This is because Anderson (1999) has many more cases of Parkinson's disease (103 vs. 31).

The meta-analysis techniques allow for the weight of each study. The simplest method is:

$$\text{Combined effect size} = \frac{\text{sum of} \left(\text{effect size} \times \text{weight for each study}\right)}{\text{sum of all the weights}}$$

Relative risk, OR, or hazard ratio (are used on a $\log_e$ scale, and the result is antilogged).

This method is called a **fixed effects model** and is the one used in Figure 10.2 (indicated by the word 'fixed' in the heading of the far right column).

The combined analysis is based on 1114 cases of Parkinson's disease and 130,477 unaffected participants; both are reasonably large, and much greater than any individual study. The combined OR is 0.81 shown as the large diamond in the row labelled 'total' in Figure 10.2. People with moderate/high vitamin E intake were 19% less likely to have Parkinson's disease than those with the lowest intake, and the true effect could be as low as a 2% decrease or as high as a 33% decrease. The 95% CI range is narrower than in any individual study, a common feature of meta-analyses. The p-value associated with the combined estimate is 0.03 (given in the row labelled 'test for overall effect'), which indicates that the OR of 0.81 is statistically significant and unlikely to be due to chance. However, the evidence is not overly strong because the p-value is not very small.

Heterogeneity

No two studies in a systematic review are identical in design and conduct, so it is necessary to consider whether the observed effect sizes materially differ from each other, that is, whether there is **heterogeneity** [16]. If they are very different, it might not be appropriate to combine the results into a single number. Figure 10.4 illustrates this concept using four hypothetical studies. Studies 1–3 appear similar (no heterogeneity), but Study 4 clearly looks different from the other three (evidence of heterogeneity). Statistical tests can help to quantify whether significant heterogeneity is present and, if it is, statistical methods can combine the effect sizes to allow for it [2].

In Figure 10.2, a **test for heterogeneity** (shown in the bottom left-hand corner, chi-squared test) produced a p-value of 0.61, suggesting that the OR estimates do not differ substantially,[#] and an appropriate method to combine the results is, therefore, a **fixed effects model**. If there is significant heterogeneity (i.e. the p-value for the test is <0.05), a **random effects model** may be more appropriate, because this method takes into account variability in the effect sizes between studies. 'Fixed' would be replaced by 'random' in the forest plot. The two methods tend to produce similar effect sizes and CIs when there is little or no heterogeneity. When there is significant heterogeneity, the

---

[#] The test actually assesses whether the individual effect sizes differ much from the combined estimate, but it is perhaps easier to think about differences between each other; and little is lost by this.

Study

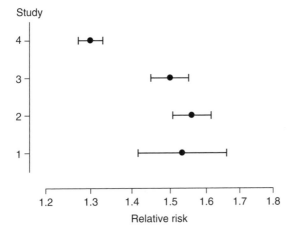

Figure 10.4 Illustration of heterogeneity among four hypothetical studies. The results from Studies 1 to 3 are similar, but the result from Study 4 is clearly different from the other three.

pooled effect sizes may still be similar, but the 'random effects' approach produces wider CIs, to allow for the between-study variability. There is more uncertainty over the size of the true effect, given the greater variability.

The standard test for heterogeneity is not very good at detecting differences between studies when there are few of them. In such circumstances, the I^2 **value** may be preferred. Using this value, 0% indicates no heterogeneity, and 100% a high degree of heterogeneity [16]. In Figure 10.2, I^2 is 0%, which is very low. In this example, the conclusion based on I^2 is consistent with the test for heterogeneity.

If significant heterogeneity is found, it should always be investigated, because the pooled effect may not be meaningful. When heterogeneity can be explained by a particular factor (e.g. age), the effect size in each subgroup of the factor describes the association better than the overall estimate. Figure 10.5 is an example, based on a meta-analysis of 13 case–control studies examining the association between mobile phone use and the risk of cancer (mainly brain) [17]. The pooled OR is 1.18, a small/modest 18% increase in risk for long-term mobile phone users (≥ 10 years). However, the test for heterogeneity is significant ($p = 0.021$), and the I^2 value is quite high (33.1%), indicating that the ORs differ. The researchers investigated this, and separated the studies according to whether or not the case/control status of the participant was known to the person collecting the data on exposures in each of the studies (i.e. whether blinding was used). When there was no blinding, there was no evidence of an association (OR 0.99 and $I^2 = 0$), but for studies with blinding, there was a 35% excess risk, which was statistically significant, though there was still evidence of heterogeneity between them ($I^2 = 35.1\%$). A further potential issue in this meta-analysis was that all the studies using blinding were conducted by the same research group (same lead author).

Researchers sometimes incorrectly assume that using a random effects model is sufficient to overcome heterogeneity. However, such an analysis cannot identify the *reasons* for heterogeneity, which can only be found by a proper and detailed assessment of the studies.

Allowing for bias and confounding

Meta-analyses of randomised trials are less affected by confounding and bias than those of observational studies, because their effects have been minimised by the process of randomisation in each trial and, where possible, by blinding of the interventions. In contrast, if one observational study is affected by confounding and bias, which produce a spurious association, the combination of several observational studies, all affected by the same issues, would compound (magnify) their effects and lead to a false but 'precise' estimate of the effect size and possibly misleading conclusions [18]. Although confounding factors, when they have been measured, could be taken into account in the analysis from each individual study, bias is more difficult to address. Determining whether major biases are present, and the likely impact on the effect size, can usually only be considered in a qualitative way, and it may not be easy to adjust the combined effect size for them.

In the example in Figure 10.5, all of the studies had a case–control design and may therefore have been affected by similar biases, such as recall and selection bias, which could have produced an association when one really did not exist. Only one study was individually statistically significant (Hardell 2006),[#] so for each of the others, it would be difficult to make a robust conclusion about the association. Combining all the studies produced an OR of only 1.18 (for ≥ 10 years use), and this could have arisen by magnifying the effect of the two biases. This could also apply to studies using blinding (Figure 10.5), which appears to produce a stronger association (OR of 1.35, with fairly narrow 95% CI). Additional evidence on this topic comes from prospective cohort studies, but their findings are inconsistent to those from case–control studies. For example, one of the largest cohort studies on the subject (358,403 participants, including 10,729 tumours of the central nervous system) [19] showed no evidence of an association with using mobile phones for ≥ 13 years: relative risk 1.03 (95% CI 0.83–1.27) among men and 0.91 (95% CI 0.41–2.04) among women. Although the upper limits allow the possibility of an excess risk, the point estimates do not. It is possible, therefore, that case–control and cohort studies produce different results due to bias or confounding, and further evidence is required before making firm conclusions about a causal link between mobile phone use and cancer.

It is, therefore, important to combine effect sizes that have already been adjusted for potential confounders, and, where possible, bias has been minimised (or at least addressed). Many studies report both unadjusted and adjusted effect sizes in their results, and different studies adjust for different potential

---

[#] Individual references are provided in the systematic review [17].

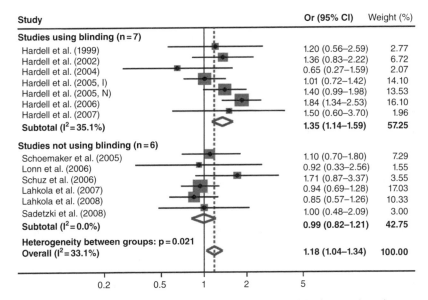

Study	Or (95% CI)	Weight (%)
Studies using blinding (n = 7)		
Hardell et al. (1999)	1.20 (0.56–2.59)	2.77
Hardell et al. (2002)	1.36 (0.83–2.22)	6.72
Hardell et al. (2004)	0.65 (0.27–1.59)	2.07
Hardell et al. (2005, I)	1.01 (0.72–1.42)	14.10
Hardell et al. (2005, N)	1.40 (0.99–1.98)	13.53
Hardell et al. (2006)	1.84 (1.34–2.53)	16.10
Hardell et al. (2007)	1.50 (0.60–3.70)	1.96
Subtotal (I^2 = 35.1%)	**1.35 (1.14–1.59)**	**57.25**
Studies not using blinding (n = 6)		
Schoemaker et al. (2005)	1.10 (0.70–1.80)	7.29
Lonn et al. (2006)	0.92 (0.33–2.56)	1.55
Schuz et al. (2006)	1.71 (0.87–3.37)	3.55
Lahkola et al. (2007)	0.94 (0.69–1.28)	17.03
Lahkola et al. (2008)	0.85 (0.57–1.26)	10.33
Sadetzki et al. (2008)	1.00 (0.48–2.09)	3.00
Subtotal (I^2 = 0.0%)	**0.99 (0.82–1.21)**	**42.75**
Heterogeneity between groups: p = 0.021		
Overall (I^2 = 33.1%)	**1.18 (1.04–1.34)**	**100.00**

0.2   0.5   1   2   5

Figure 10.5 Forest plot of mobile phone use of ≥ 10 years and the risk of cancer, based on a meta-analysis of 13 case–control studies [16], according to whether the interviewer (researcher) who obtained information from the participants (including exposure status) was blinded or not to their case–control status. Source: Myung et al., 2009 [17]. Reproduced by permission of the American Society of Clinical Oncology.

confounders. The following approaches could be taken when conducting a meta-analysis of observational studies:

• Check whether each study has considered important confounders.
• Use the adjusted estimates, and use unadjusted estimates only when the adjusted effect sizes are unavailable.
• Perform an additional meta-analysis (could be called a **sensitivity analysis**) using only the adjusted effect sizes, to see how this compares with the meta-analysis based on all estimates (adjusted and unadjusted). Does the effect size diminish when focussing only on the adjusted estimates?

Sensitivity Analysis

Figure 10.6 is a forest plot using studies summarised in Table 10.2, examining the association between women who smoke during pregnancy and the risk of having a baby with a limb defect [13]. A sensitivity analysis could examine subgroups of studies, to look for consistency. For example, the combined OR was 1.26 (95% CI 1.15–1.39) for all eight studies (26% higher risk among women who smoked), but some studies did not make any adjustment for potential confounding factors (i.e. Kallen 2000, Robitaille 2009, Table 10.2).#

Individual references are provided in the systematic review [13].

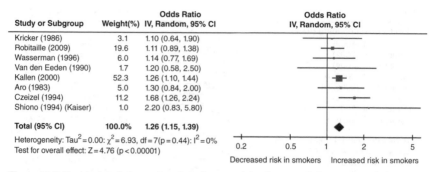

Figure 10.6 Forest plot of observational studies examining the association between maternal smoking and the risk of limb reduction defects in babies. Data from Ref [13].

By restricting the meta-analysis to those that did (Aro 1983, Kricker 1986, Van Den Eeden 1990, Czeizel 1994, and Wasserman 1996), the pooled OR becomes 1.37 (95% CI 1.14–1.65), which is higher than the overall value of 1.26. In two studies (Shiono 1986 and Wasserman 1996), the authors examined the adjusted ORs but did not provide them in the published paper, stating only that they were 'similar' to the unadjusted ones. Even if Wasserman (1996) were excluded (confounding was only considered as matching factors, rather than actual adjustments in the statistical analysis), the pooled OR in the remaining four studies still shows an excess risk: 1.44, 95% CI 1.17–1.78. These observations are consistent with Figure 10.6, because the studies produce similar ORs, despite differences in weights. It is also reassuring that even when the study with the largest weight (Kallen 2000, 52.3%) is excluded, the pooled effect sizes are not too dissimilar.

10.5 Considerations when reading a systematic review

There are several aspects of any review to consider when deciding whether it provides good evidence for, or against, an association.

Differences in disease definition, the exposures, and outcome measures

Studies are conducted in different ways using a variety of methods, and the definition of the exposures and the outcome measures may all vary between studies. In the studies in Figure 10.2, the comparison group consisted of participants who had the lowest dietary consumption of vitamin E, and the definition of 'low' will vary between different populations. It is not always easily possible to combine studies in a systematic review, particularly if the designs are very different. However, if different studies produce similar results, this may itself provide some evidence of an association, because the difference in methodology should increase variability, making it more difficult to find a relationship between an exposure and outcome measure. When deciding whether a study should be included in a review it is also useful to determine whether the chosen endpoints are appropriate for addressing the review objective, and this may be influenced by studies that did or did not use standard/established methods for diagnosing the disorder of interest.

Identifying studies

Systematic review reports should provide sufficient information on how studies were identified, by specifying the search criteria employed. This information includes the range of years over which articles were published, whether foreign language articles were excluded, and which databases were used (e.g. Medline and Embase). The choice of appropriate keywords is fundamental when searching databases. In a review of a risk factor for cancer, it is insufficient to search using only the word 'cancer'; some abstracts may use 'tumour' or 'carcinoma'. There are also different spellings e.g. 'tumor' and different variations of the same words e.g. 'prospective' and 'prospectively'. Wildcards are useful, the search term would be 'prospective'*, where the asterisk allows for any letters after 'prospective'. If studies are missed, the review may not be representative, and the results could be biased. Authors of systematic reviews often provide a flow diagram of the study identification process, showing how the final set of studies included in the meta-analysis was derived from the initial search of the electronic databases. An example for the review of mobile phone use and cancer is shown in Figure 10.7.

Publication bias

There is evidence that studies with 'negative' results (those contrary to what is expected or those reporting no evidence of an effect) are less likely to be published than those showing an effect, either because the research is not submitted for publication or because journals favour papers showing 'successful' studies and therefore reject them [20–22]. When this occurs, the pooled effect size from the meta-analysis will be biased towards the positive studies, and will, therefore, be larger than the true value. A simple statistical method that can detect significant publication bias is a **funnel plot**, which plots the effect size against the weight, represented as any of the following: standard error, 1/standard error, or 1/standard error^2. If the spread of the observations is clearly asymmetric, this is evidence of possible publication bias [23]. Figure 10.8 is a funnel plot for the studies of vitamin E and Parkinson's disease. The hypothesis is that vitamin E could be protective, so publication bias would appear as noticeable gaps in the right hand side of the figure (where ORs of ≥ 1 indicate no association or that high dietary intake increases risk), which is not the case here. However, while there is no clear asymmetry to the observations, there are perhaps too few studies to make a reliable assessment of publication bias.

Study quality

Study quality may be discussed, and those judged to be inferior excluded from the meta-analysis.

Exclusion could be based on an assessment of the study design, conduct, or analysis, and consideration of whether or not potential bias or confounding have been satisfactorily addressed. Criteria for inclusion could include appropriate definition or diagnosis of people with the disorder (or event) of interest,

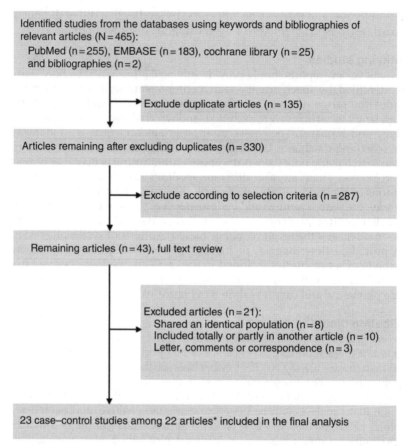

*one article was divided into two studies because it included two different tumour types

Figure 10.7 Flow diagram showing how the case–control studies for the meta-analysis of mobile phone use and cancer were identified (see Figure 10.5). Source: Myung et al., 2009 [15]. Reproduced by permission of the American Society of Clinical Oncology.

appropriate measures of the exposures, and use of blinding when making assessments or collecting data. Even if the criteria for exclusion are clearly defined, this is a subjective exercise that could itself produce a biased selection of studies to be used in the meta-analysis.

Different study designs (cross-sectional, case–control, and cohort) can influence the assessment of quality. If there are enough studies in the review, an attempt could be made to combine the effect sizes according to each design, and compare the findings for consistency (or inconsistency).

If a study is affected by bias or confounding, consideration should be given to whether their influence is so great that they clearly distort the results. When assessing the effect of study quality, it is perhaps best to include all studies in

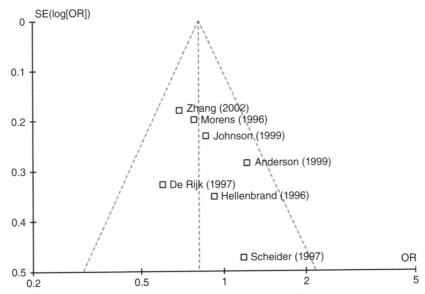

Figure 10.8 Funnel plot of the seven studies of Parkinson's disease shown in Figure 10.2. The x-axis is the odds OR, and the y-axis is the standard error based. The vertical line is the combined effect size (0.81). Small studies, with large standard errors, could be more likely to have large effects. Therefore, publication bias may be present if the funnel plot shows a very asymmetric pattern. Source: Etminan et al., 2012 [13]. Reproduced by permission of Elsevier.

an initial meta-analysis and then perform a meta-analysis after excluding those considered 'poor quality'. Results can be compared to assess consistency (another form of **sensitivity analysis**).

10.6 Reporting systematic reviews

The methodology employed in systematic reviews must be reported clearly, so that health professionals can judge the reliability of the results and conclusions. A report based on a systematic review should include the following items (a more detailed set of guidelines can be found elsewhere [24]):

- The main objective.
- The search strategy, including the search terms and electronic databases used, as well as other sources of studies.
- The inclusion criteria for full articles selected for the meta-analysis, including specification of the target population, the disorder, the exposures, and the endpoints.
- The total number of abstracts found during the electronic search, how many full articles were examined, how many were used in the meta-analysis, how many were excluded, and the reasons for their exclusion.
- A table summarising the main characteristics of each study used in the meta-analysis, such as geographical location, time period when the study

was conducted, sample size, key features of the individuals (e.g. age range and gender distribution), the exposure, outcome measure, the effect size used, and confounding factors allowed for.
• Method of meta-analysis (fixed or random effects model) and any investigation of heterogeneity if it exists such as a formal statistical test or I^2 value should be provided.
• Specifying the implications for clinical practice or knowledge should be discussed, including recommendations for further studies if appropriate.

10.7 Key points

• Systematic reviews are based on a formal approach to obtaining, analysing, and interpreting all the available studies on a particular topic.
• A meta-analysis combines all relevant studies to give a single estimate of the effect size, which has greater precision than any individual study.
• The conclusions from a review are usually stronger than those from any single study.
• However, reviews at observational studies could magnify the effect of common biases or confounders, producing a spurious association with precise estimates of effect size.
• Any noticeable heterogeneity as well as the presence of significant confounding and bias must be properly investigated and discussed.

References

1. Glasziou P, Irwig L, Bain C, Colditz G. Systematic Reviews in Health Care: A Practical Guide. Cambridge University Press (2001).
2. Khan KS, Kunz R, Kleijnen J, Antes G. Systematic Reviews to Support Evidence-based Medicine: How to Review and Apply Findings of Healthcare Research. Royal Society of Medicine Press (2003).
3. Egger M, Davey SG, Altman D. Systematic Reviews in Health Care: Meta-analysis in Context. WileyBlackwell. Second Edition (2001).
4. Egger M, Davey SG. Meta-analysis: potentials and promise. BMJ 1997;315:1371–4.
5. Egger M, Davey SG, Phillips AN. Meta-analysis: principles and procedures. BMJ 1997;315:1533–7.
6. Davey SG, Egger M, Phillips AN. Meta-analysis: beyond the grand mean? BMJ 1997;315:1610–14.
7. Hirayama T. Cancer mortality in nonsmoking women with smoking husbands based on a large-scale cohort study in Japan. Prev Med 1984;13(6):680–90.
8. Wu-Williams AH, Dai XD, Blot W, Xu ZY, Sun XW, Xiao HP, et al. Lung cancer among women in north-east China. Br J Cancer 1990;62(6):982–7.
9. Enstrom JE, Kabat GC. Environmental tobacco smoke and tobacco related mortality in a prospective study of Californians, 1960–98. BMJ 2003;326(7398):1057.
10. Puntoni R, Toninelli F, Zhankui L, Bonassi S. Mathematical modelling in risk/exposure assessment of tobacco related lung cancer. Carcinogenesis 1995;16:1465–71.
11. Hackshaw AK, Law MR, Wald NJ. The accumulated evidence on lung cancer and environmental tobacco smoke. BMJ 1997;315(7114):980–8.

12. Wald NJ, Nanchahal K, Thompson SG, Cuckle HS. Does breathing other people's tobacco smoke cause lung cancer? BMJ 1986;293(6556):1217–22.
13. Hackshaw A, Rodeck C, Boniface S. Maternal smoking in pregnancy and birth defects: a systematic review based on 173 687 malformed cases and 11.7 million controls. Hum Reprod Update 2011;17(5):589–604.
14. Etminan M, Gill SS, Samii A. Intake of vitamin E, vitamin C, and carotenoids and the risk of Parkinson's disease: a meta-analysis. Lancet Neurol 2005;4(6):362–5.
15. Review Manager (RevMan) [Computer program]. Version 5.1. The Nordic Cochrane Centre, The Cochrane Collaboration (2011).
16. Higgins JPT, Thompson SG, Deeks JJ, Altman DG. Measuring inconsistency in meta-analyses. BMJ 2003;327:557–60.
17. Myung SK, Ju W, McDonnell DD, Lee YJ, Kazinets G, Cheng CT, Moskowitz JM. Mobile phone use and risk of tumors: a meta-analysis. J Clin Oncol 2009;27(33):5565–72.
18. Egger M, Schneider M, Davey SG. Meta-analysis: spurious precision? Meta-analysis of observational studies. BMJ 1998;316:140–4.
19. Frei P, Poulsen AH, Johansen C, Olsen JH, Steding-Jessen M, Schüz J. Use of mobile phones and risk of brain tumours: update of Danish cohort study. BMJ 2011;343:d6387. doi:10.1136/bmj.d6387.
20. Sterne JAC, Egger M, Davey SG. Systematic reviews in health care: investigating and dealing with publication and other biases in meta-analysis. BMJ 2001;323:101–5.
21. Egger M, Davey SG. Meta-analysis: bias in location and selection of studies. BMJ 1998;316:61–6.
22. Jannot AS, Agoritsas T, Gayet-Ageron A, Perneger TV. Citation bias favoring statistically significant studies was present in medical research. J Clin Epidemiol. 2013;66(3):296–301.
23. Egger M, Davey SG, Schneider M, Minder CE. Bias in meta-analysis detected by a simple graphical test. BMJ 1997;315:629–4.
24. von Elm E, Altman DG, Egger M, Pocock SJ, Gøtzsche PC, Vandenbroucke JP; STROBE Initiative. The Strengthening the Reporting of Observational Studies in Epidemiology (STROBE) statement: guidelines for reporting observational studies. Ann Intern Med 2007;147(8):573–7.

CHAPTER 11

Conducting and reporting observational studies

There are established systems for conducting and reporting observational studies, and most will proceed through a standard set of stages (Box 11.1).

11.1 Before conducting the study

Establishing a working group and a study team

A small multidisciplinary **working group** of key people (perhaps three to five, but possibly more) should initially develop the project. The group could include relevant health professionals, a statistician, and other members with specialist backgrounds.

After securing funding, the group can expand to form the **study team** (sometimes also called **study management group**, or **study steering group/ committee**) to manage the project over its entire duration. This team could additionally include expertise in data management, regulations and safety monitoring, IT (database systems). It is also worth including potential collaborators, especially recruiting centres from which either participants or data will be obtained.

Estimate the financial costs of the study

The cost of conducting an observational study varies; small-scale studies, which only involve retrieving data from medical records within a single department or institution, may not incur costs if the researcher is already a member of staff and conducts the project as part of their work. However, multicentre studies, in which participants are recruited and followed up for several months or years, can be expensive to set up and conduct and so require staff to co-ordinate the project. The number and type of staff required will depend on the complexity of the study and sample size, and could include staff to perform and provide any of the following:

- Participant recruitment
- Retrieving data from medical records
- Study co-ordination (set-up, conduct, and close down, including dealing with queries from sites and possibly participants)

A Concise Guide to Observational Studies in Healthcare, First Edition. Allan Hackshaw.
© 2015 John Wiley & Sons, Ltd. Published 2015 by John Wiley & Sons, Ltd.

Box 11.1 Elements to a typical process for conducting an observational study (not all apply to all studies)

Pre-study

Establish working group to develop idea.
Identify and approach potential collaborators/sites.
Estimate the financial costs.
Secure grant funding.

Study set-up

Develop protocol, Participant Information Sheet (PIS), consent form, and questionnaires.
Obtain ethical or institutional review board (IRB) approval.
Develop the case report forms (CRFs) and database.
Develop any necessary agreements and contracts.
Obtain approval from each site.
Set-up study in centres (e.g. site assessment and initiation).
Activate sites.

Conduct study

Develop standard operating procedures (SOPs).
Regular meetings of the research team.
Monitor progress in sites (including adverse events).
Independent Data Monitoring Committee (IDMC) review.
Send annual progress report to ethics committee/IRB.

End of study

Final checks of database.
Inform ethics committee of study closure.
Sponsor and recruiting sites should store all relevant documentation.
Publish results.
Long-term follow-up.

- Data management (e.g. data entry and checking)
- Development and maintenance of a study-specific database, or collating electronic data from different database systems
- Collecting and processing biological samples
- Statistical support
- Pathology services
- Administration and collection of data forms

The salary costs for these staff will depend on the time they are expected to spend on the study and where the work will be undertaken (central research unit or recruitment at centres).

Other direct costs to consider include:
- Those to be met by recruiting centres: for example, extra clinical assessments, data collection and recording, extra blood or tissue sampling, extra imaging scans, or laboratory analyses.

• Office and travel expenses, printing protocols and case report forms (see page 226), travel and other costs for the research group meetings, and setting up centres and visits to them during the study.
• Applications to the independent ethics committee (see page 225).
• Cost of flagging participants for deaths (or other disorders, such as cancer) with regional or national registries.
• A payment made to each participant recruited especially if they have to complete long detailed questionnaires or face-to-face interviews; this is usually only done for relatively small observational studies and is essentially a payment for the 'inconvenience' in taking part in the study.
• Payments to participants for travel and/or subsistence expenses for extra clinic visits.
• Cost of consumables and equipment (including fridges or freezers) for collecting and storing biological samples for translational research.

Grant funding

Grants to conduct observational studies are limited and competitive, and they usually come from governmental bodies, research councils, charities, or private benefactors. Pharmaceutical companies do not often provide grants for observational studies. However, many academic departments are able to run small- or even moderate-sized observational studies without external funding, and studies based on data already collected should require minimal resources, if any (perhaps only for the statistical analysis and some IT input).

The previous section covered direct costs attributed to the study, but for institutions such as universities, there can be overheads (indirect costs) that need to be added to the grant. These costs are meant to cover central support and administrative resources, used by staff conducting the study who are employed by the institution.

Figure 11.1 shows the main items to address in a typical grant application. Funding bodies seek value for money and are likely to only support studies that have the potential to change practice or that involve novel translational research. If funding is to be sought, the key issues of the application should be considered thoroughly by the working group to ensure that there are no oversights or errors that could be picked up for the first time by the funding committee or their external reviewers. Although the format of the application forms will vary between funding organisations, many aspects are often covered by the study protocol[#] (see page 219). Further details about how to develop grant applications can be found elsewhere [1].

11.2 Study set-up

Some research departments have the primary purpose to design, set up, and analyse studies involving humans, and so should have permanent staff in place, often including clinicians, health professionals, statisticians, co-ordinators,

---

[#] Formal protocols are not always required by a funding organisation as a part of grant application

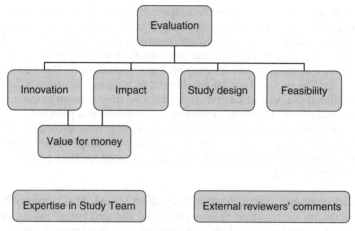

Figure 11.1 Key aspects of a typical grant application used by a funding committee for evaluation purposes.

data managers, and IT/database staff. Having access to such departments is important for large-scale studies, particularly if they involve following up the study participants.

Potential recruiting centres, sometimes referred to as a **site**, should be identified, with a realistic estimate of the number of expected participants per site (investigators tend to overestimate this). This helps ensure that the target sample size is feasible in a reasonable time frame.

Sponsor, lead study researcher, and other investigators

A sponsor is the institution with ultimate responsibility for the design and conduct of the study. The concept of a sponsor is often only used for studies that involve recruiting participants and obtaining information (including biological samples) directly from them, and also when they are to be followed up for several months or years. Studies using data already collected probably do not need a sponsor, but local guidelines should be checked on this.

The **chief investigator** is the lead researcher for the study and often first developed the idea. A Principal Investigator (**PI**) is an individual responsible for the study at a single recruiting centre, so a multicentre study would have several PIs. These are not standard labels, but their roles often are. A chief investigator is sometimes called a PI.

Study protocol

A protocol should be developed for any study that involves recruiting participants. It may be required as part of a grant application submission, otherwise it must be developed before application for ethical approval is made. It provides a summary of the justification for the study, details of the design, and a set of instructions for sites and (if applicable) the co-ordinating centre, describing how participants are to be recruited (including eligibility) and followed up. It should provide the basis to ensure that the study is conducted to a similar standard across all sites. Studies that do not involve direct contact with participants (e.g. those only using data to be extracted from medical records) might still benefit from having a (usually much shorter) protocol, focussing on the study design and analysis. The protocol can be any length, as long as it contains a clear plan of what will happen to participants, from the time they consent to the time they leave the study. Box 11.2 shows suggested key sections in a protocol.

An important part of the protocol is describing how biological samples should be collected, processed, and stored. If this is not specified in the protocol, there should be an Standard Operating Procedure that provides these details (see page 231).

Informed consent, participant information sheet, and consent form

All participants are required to give **informed consent** before taking part for many observational studies. This includes studies where people are:

- To be interviewed or to complete questionnaires
- Asked to donate biological samples for research purposes, either taken during usual clinical practice or specific to the study
- To be followed up over time and data collected from them or their medical records
- Asked to undergo study-specific assessments, for example, physical examinations or imaging (e.g. X-rays), that they would not normally have in routine practice
- At risk of suffering physical or psychological harm by being in the study

Depending on local regulations and guidelines, there are studies in which informed consent may not be required, such as those using only data from medical records, or stored biological samples (often linked with clinical data). Indeed, there is evidence that if informed consent were obtained in studies like these, the characteristics of those who agree to participate differ from those who do not, creating a bias in the study outcome measures and results [2]. Also, there are some studies where obtaining consent from each participant is not possible or feasible. In others, where people are asked to complete a questionnaire, those who do so have implicitly consented. In these situations, although participants are not asked directly to take part, there should still be an independent review and approval of the project by an independent ethics committee (see page 225), who will stipulate whether or not participants' consent is required.

When informed consent is required, sufficient information about the study must be provided to allow potential participants to understand the objectives and examine the possible benefits and risks of taking part. Information may be provided verbally, but it is usually given as a leaflet: the **Participant Information Sheet (PIS)**. After reading this, participants sign and date a **consent form**, which is co-signed by an authorised staff member. Suggested sections are shown in Boxes 11.3 and 11.4. Signed consent forms should be kept in the site files, and a copy given to the participant. Sometimes, signed forms are not appropriate, for

Box 11.2 Sections in a study protocol (not all sections apply to all studies)

Heading	Description
Chief investigator and Sponsor	• Name and address of the lead individual, and the sponsor's representative
Study management	• Names, affiliations, and roles of the research team
Background and justification	• Concise summary of the disorder/topic, and its scale (e.g. prevalence or incidence), including biological plausibility, and why the study is needed
Objectives (hypotheses)	• Clear specification of the aims (simple language)
Study Design	• Cross-sectional, case-control, retrospective or prospective cohort
Exposures	• Should be listed and well-defined, including how they are to be measured
Outcome measures	• Each objective should be associated with a quantifiable outcome measure; including how they are to be measured
Sample size	• Include enough information for the sample size to be reproduced independently, with justification of the expected effect
Target population	• Inclusion and exclusion criteria, and describe the sampling frame
Consent and approvals	• Procedures for obtaining informed consent, and ethics/institutional approvals
Assessment of participants; data collection	• Details of how participants will be assessed, including how frequently, and what will happen at each visit (e.g. clinical examinations) • Whether extra clinic visits are needed in addition to usual care • Describe how data are to be collected: • Self-completed questionnaires (and how the researchers can collect these) • Face-to-face interviews (how these would be organised) • Retrieving data from hospital/clinic records, regional or national databases/registries • Procedures for collecting, storing, and processing biological samples, including posting conditions, and any specialist equipment required
Recruitment and Follow up	• Expected length of total accrual, and follow up for each participant.
Safety monitoring	• List of potential harms, and procedures for identifying, monitoring, and reporting them
Statistical analyses	• The main statistical methods to be used
Insurance and indemnity	• Details of what cover is in place if a participant is harmed through participating in the study
Ownership & publication	• A statement about ownership of the study data, and authorship of any publications that arise from the study

---

Box 11.3 Recommended sections in a Participant Information Sheet (PIS)

• Background and justification for the study.
• Why the participant has been invited to take part.
• What the participant has to do as part of the study (e.g. self-completed question-naires, interviews, attend clinic for assessments) and the expected duration of their participation.
• Which biological samples, if any, are being collected and what will be done with them for the purpose of the study.* It could be mentioned that the samples will be stored for future research, which may include genetic testing.
• If blood or urine samples are to be taken, make clear how much (in scientific units such as millilitres, in addition to using simpler measures such as the number of teaspoons).
• What are the possible harms of being in the study.
• The possible benefits and disadvantages of taking part.
• A statement about securing confidentiality of data and who will have access to the data.
• A description of using regional or national registry data (e.g. death registries, cancer occurrences) and an explanation that the participant would need to be flagged (linked or tracked) via the registry, which may require personal identifiers such as full name and national identification numbers.**
• A statement that participation is voluntary and refusal to participate will involve no penalty or loss of benefit and that the participant may withdraw at any time.
• Who is funding the research.
• Who to contact during the study if there are any queries or if there is a problem.
• A statement about liability and compensation if something goes wrong.

*Some PISs state that samples are to be stored in a particular institution. This should probably be avoided because if the samples need to move to another institution later on (for whatever reason) researchers would want to avoid having to send out a revised PIS to all participants and re-consent them just on this aspect.
**Consent for using these identifiers should be specifically requested on the consent form.

---

example, studies of sensitive issues such as taking illicit drugs or sexual habits, because anonymity is needed. Consent may also be obtained by telephone, if this is how data are to be collected anyway.

If a potential participant is unable to provide informed consent, for example, children or incapacitated adults, a guardian or representative (usually a parent, or other close relative) could be asked instead. This must be made clear in the application for independent ethics review.

Anonymity is an important feature of research (i.e. individual participants cannot be identified by researchers, nor should they be identifiable in publica-tions), and it should be specified in the PIS. Participant names or initial with dates of birth should not be used routinely. However, if the researchers require person identifiers (e.g. full name, address, national identification numbers, initials, and date of birth), this must be specifically requested on the consent form (Box 11.4). For example, there are studies with regular questionnaires (e.g. yearly) to be posted to participants, so full contact details are essential to

---

Box 11.4 Example of text used in a consent form

• I confirm that I have read and understand the information sheet dated 15 March 2013 version 3.0. I have had the opportunity to consider the information, ask questions, and have had these answered satisfactorily.

• I understand that my participation is voluntary and that I am free to withdraw at any time, without giving any reason and without my medical care or legal rights being affected.

• I understand that relevant sections of any of my medical notes and data collected during the study may be looked at by appropriate individuals from the institution(s) involved in this research or from relevant regulatory bodies.

• I agree to my family physician being informed of my participation in this study and that they may be contacted to supply details of my progress.

• I agree to give blood samples, urine samples, and diagnostic tissue samples for research purposes. I understand how these samples will be taken, and that my participation is voluntary. I am free to withdraw my approval for their use at any time without giving a reason and without my medical treatment or legal rights being affected. I can request that any samples stored by the research team that can still be identified as mine should be destroyed.

• I agree that the blood/tissue samples I have given and the information gathered about me can be stored for use in future research studies

• I consent to the collection of personal information (including my initials, date of birth and gender) for the purposes of this study. I understand that any information that could identify me will be kept strictly confidential and that no personal information will be included in any publication

• I agree to participate in the study

Signature of the study subject or legal guardian   ....

Signature of researcher   ....

---

the study. There are often clear local guidelines or regulations regarding **data protection** and **confidentiality**.

The text in the PIS and consent form should be written in simple language. It is often useful to ask a few potential participants, lay people, members of a patient representative group or research nurse, to comment on the text before it is finalised, particularly for complex studies. This is because they may read and interpret the PIS differently from the researchers.

There are studies in which a previously undiagnosed disorder is found in a participant. If this disorder is among the study objectives, then it is appropriate that the result is sent to the participant and his/her family physician, and the procedures for this should be specified in the protocol and the PIS. If the disorder is unrelated to the study objectives (i.e. an incidental finding), the issue requires consideration, particularly when it is one that should be treated. Further investigations, with possible interventions, would not be part of the study protocol, but if the disorder can be readily linked to the participant, then it is appropriate to inform them, usually through their family physician, after which they can seek standard care outside of the study.

Genetic testing using donated biological specimens is becoming more common. It may be done among healthy participants (e.g. general population) or those who already have a disorder (e.g. cancer patients). However, there are potential issues with this regarding what information, if any, is reported back to participants. Finding a 'high risk' gene or genetic mutation is possible, but the researchers must carefully consider whether it is one that is established to be correlated with a disorder (or other outcomes such as early death). There will be many mutations for which the clinical implications are as yet unknown, and there may even be consequences for health insurance. Offering genetic results to participant's (in prospective studies) may be recommended, when all of the following four conditions hold [3]:

1. There is established analytic validity (the laboratory testing is reliable, with appropriate quality control).
2. The association between the gene or mutation and the disorder is replicable and clinically significant, for example, relative risk >2.0; including significant reproductive risks for disease among offspring.
3. The disorder has important health implications, such as early death or substantial morbidity.
4. Proven therapeutic or preventive interventions are available.

If the genetic results can be readily linked to individuals, or the participants expect to be told the results, the researchers must have a system in place for reporting this information, counselling and appropriate interventions for those found to have an abnormal result. All of this will probably require funding. Furthermore, while some genetic testing may be done during or at the end of the study, some studies will only perform this in the future, so there will be ethical implications in contacting a study participant from several/many years before, regarding a detected genetic defect or high-risk gene. Finally, it is important that if genetic results are to be reported back to participants, this should be specified in both the PIS and consent form, that is, the participants need to agree to this. If genetic testing is to be kept anonymous, that is, participants are not informed, this should also be stated (example in Box 11.5).

All participants are able to withdraw their consent during the study at any time. Participants who withdraw usually do so because they no longer wish to continue with study-specific assessments, including completing questionnaires, but they may also wish to withdraw consent to use any of their data. In practice, if data are only to be extracted from their medical records, many participants who withdraw do not mind if this continues, and this option should be made clear to them at the time. Sometimes, the consent form states that the researchers will use data collected up to the point when participants withdraw, but not afterwards.

For observational studies that involve recruiting and following up participants, especially large multicentre studies, the research team could consider having a publicly accessible website (the address for which is included in the PIS). The website could have general updates about the project every 6 or 12 months, including information such as which sites (centres) are open, number of participants recruited, and general problems encountered by participants (with Frequently Asked Questions). The value of such a website would be to

> **Box 11.5 Example of text from an observational study examining molecular markers in blood and tumour tissue provided by patients with lung cancer [4]**
>
> **What is the purpose of the study?**
>
> We know that lung cancer grows and spreads, but there is much variation in how this happens. The purpose of the study is to look at biological features of lung cancers (including the genetic make-up), to see how it changes after diagnosis, and during and after treatment.
>
> **What will the samples be used for?**
>
> The tissue biopsies will be analysed for a range of genetic and non-genetic changes in the tumour, at a central research laboratory. The tissue and blood samples will also be stored for further research, to allow us to better understand lung cancer and its treatment. Any genetic testing performed on these samples will be done anonymously, and the results cannot be traced to you personally.
>
> **What will happen to any samples I give?**
>
> Any samples you provide will be given a unique identifier, and will not be able to be traced back to you. These samples will be regarded as a donation, and will be used for lung cancer research in the future.

make participants feel more involved in the study, which can encourage continuation and reduce drop outs and loss to follow-up.

If a study involves collecting biological specimens that might be used to develop a commercial product, this should be mentioned in the PIS, including a brief statement that study participants would not be able to personally benefit financially from the research.

Independent approval of the research

Many observational studies require review and approval by an **independent ethics committee** or **Institutional Review Board**. This is a group of health professionals and lay people who will examine the study protocol, and any documentation intended for participants, such as the PIS, consent form, and questionnaires, all of which are submitted via appropriate channels (and usually includes a specific application form). The process for obtaining ethical approval varies between countries, but the committee or board will consider:
- The scientific justification for and design of the study
- Acceptability to participants, including an assessment of potential harms and benefits and what clinical tests or assessments are required as part of the study
- The suitability of the investigators
- Confirm whether or not informed consent is required and, if it is, the acceptable mechanism for this

The committee may request changes to the study design, conduct, or documentation (including the PIS), and there is usually a time limit during which they must make a decision (e.g. 60 days). There is sometimes a dialogue between the researchers and the committee, if aspects of the study need to be resolved, and the committee can request further information before finalising their decision.

An application is stronger if the study has already had independent peer review, for example, through a grant application process. Involvement of lay people or patient representatives in developing the PIS and consent form could demonstrate that the wording is likely to be acceptable to potential participants.

During the study, any planned significant change to the design or conduct, particularly if it relates to how participants are recruited, assessed, or followed up, can be referred to as a **substantial amendment**. This must be submitted to the independent ethics committee or IRB for review and approval before being implemented.

Case report forms (CRFs)

In many studies, data are collected from participants. These data could come from their medical records, clinical assessments and tests performed as part of the study, or self-completed questionnaires. Data based on biological samples usually come directly from the laboratory. Study-specific case report forms (CRFs) are an efficient way of collecting some of these data. Examples of general CRFs are:

- **Baseline CRF:** Includes items such as date of entry to the study, date of birth, demographics, and perhaps information about current or past lifestyle habits and characteristics.
- **Assessment CRF:** Includes details and results of clinical assessments or tests performed as part of the study, and study-specific or established questionnaires.
- **Exposure CRF:** These are associated with measuring exposures during the study and other factors that are expected to change after baseline.
- **Outcome CRF:** Used to collect information on outcomes, such as disorders of interest (e.g. date of diagnosis and how the diagnosis was made).
- **Safety CRF:** Includes details about adverse events: type, severity, and duration.

CRFs should be simple and relatively quick to complete; achieving this objective will also reduce the time taken to enter the data onto an **electronic database**. It is important to ensure that information on the main study endpoints and confounding factors are as complete as possible, that is, with minimal missing data, and avoid collecting information that is unlikely to be used.

CRFs are often printed and completed by hand by a researcher or the participant, before the data are entered onto an electronic database. There is increasing use of **Electronic Data Capture (EDC)** systems, where staff at each site can record data directly onto the central database, via a computer, using electronic rather than paper CRFs. This minimises paperwork and should reduce time spent processing data, though there is a cost associated with developing and maintaining this type of system.

Database

Data should be stored in a well-structured and easy-to-use format, so that researchers can understand the data and perform statistical analyses easily.

All study data should be entered onto an electronic database. For small, simple studies, a spreadsheet programme such as Microsoft Excel might be acceptable. Although these programmes are easy to use, they allow data to be entered in any format, including a mixture of numbers and characters, and without any clear structure. For example, a date could be entered as '24-May-2012' or '24/05/12'; these are easy for people to read, but statistical analysis software will not accept the different formats. In practice, many Excel spreadsheets require much manual data manipulation and editing before they can be analysed, and researchers often underestimate the extent of this. If such spreadsheets are planned, it is worth being very strict about how data are entered into the columns; use simple coding where possible (e.g. 1 = male, 2 = female); and make use of drop-down fields to provide pre-specified options of which one is selected for each cell.

For multicentre or large studies, it might be better to use a commercially available (e.g. Microsoft Access) or bespoke database system. This ensures that data entry is properly structured. There are also systems that integrate a database entry facility with statistical analyses software, such as Epi Info [5] or SPSS [6]. Epi Info is free and has the most common types of statistical analyses. By using a dedicated (bespoke) database, the computer screens can be made to look similar to the paper CRFs, making data entry easier.

Automated validation checks can minimise data entry error or identify errors on the CRFs that need to be queried. For example, there could be an electronic check that the date of birth precedes the date of study registration. Range checks could be used to identify extreme blood and physiological measurements. The database could also help identify missing/incomplete data for individuals (particularly key variables) or overdue CRFs that need to be chased up.

Any database system must store data securely, with access limited to relevant research staff, especially if it contains personal identifiable information. Data should be backed up regularly, to avoid losing work if the system malfunctions.

The database must not contain any personal identifiers if the study is meant to be anonymised and participants have not given their consent to store these data.

Agreements and contracts

The extent of oversight and accountability associated with human research studies has increased over time, and one consequence is the requirement for formal agreements or contracts between institutions (governmental, academic, or commercial organisations) that are involved in the study.

The following are the main types of agreements often used. The names of the agreements may vary, and local guidelines and the sponsor will specify which are necessary and what details they need to contain. There are legal implications associated with fraud (falsifying participants or data), negligence, and lack of informed consent.

Some agreements may not be legally binding, but they aim to ensure that all parties understand the detail and standards of the work to be undertaken.

Much of the content in the documents will be standard text used by the institution (sponsor), but it is worthwhile for the chief (principal) investigator and/or other key research study members to look at and approve sections that are specific to the study. Occasionally, there could be protracted negotiations between the legal or administrative staff processing the agreements at the two institutions, and guidance from the study team could quickly clarify issues, and determine the importance of study-specific aspects of the agreements.

Clinical study site agreement
This type of agreement may be used when the observational study involves recruiting participants (or perhaps retrieving data) from several sites and is between the sponsor (often the co-ordinating centre) and each site from which participants or data are to be obtained. It should list the roles and responsibilities of the sponsor, the site, and the PI at the site. It aims to ensure that each site conducts the study according to appropriate standards, and that all data are sent to the co-ordinating centre. It also specifies the sponsor's responsibilities, for example, appropriate data management and ensuring that the site is always informed of any relevant documentation and revisions. If part of the study protocol is incorrect, a site may claim compensation from the sponsor if, for example, a participant has suffered harm as a consequence. Similarly, the sponsor may claim compensation from the site if, for example, participants or data have been falsified. The agreement should state the amount of money to which each claim is limited.

Material transfer agreement
If biological specimens are to be sent from a recruiting site to a central laboratory or biobank for specific or future research, an agreement is usually required between the site and destination organisation, to ensure that, for example, samples are handled safely and stored appropriately. The sponsor may also wish to have a service agreement with the central depository, to clarify the roles and responsibility of each party in relation to the biological samples. If the central laboratory is within the sponsor organisation, items in this agreement could be included in the clinical study site agreement, rather than have a separate one.

Technical or service-level agreements
These agreements may be needed between the sponsor (or the main institution in which the research team is based) and any third-party institution or organisation providing services for the study, such as storage or laboratory analyses of biological samples, pathology reviews, and IT or statistical support, if any of these are outsourced. Box 11.6 lists the potential items to be included in such an agreement.

Intellectual property
It is sometimes thought that the study participant ultimately 'owns' their data and samples and can withdraw their consent to use them. However, the sponsor (or research team) are the custodians of the dataset and biobank. Any

---

Box 11.6   Main items that may be included in an agreement between a study sponsor (research team) and a third party providing a service for the study

- Assurance that the third party has the necessary licenses, authorisations, or procedures in place to perform the work
- Details of the scope of the work, for example, the specific analyses to be performed, and that additional projects or analyses cannot be performed without prior agreement of the sponsor or research team
- An undertaking that any major changes to the agreed procedures, as well as any major technical problems, should be reported to the sponsor or research team
- Agreement to keep data and other findings confidential
- Whether or not the third party needs to review any publication of the results before they are submitted to a conference or journal and, if so, the length of the time for the review
- Conditions for terminating the agreement
- How payments are to be paid

---

intellectual property (IP) rights directly arising from the research should be made clear, when there are several collaborators, and the potential for identifying new technologies, or new biological and genetic markers for health outcomes, using patentable methods. If one institution sponsors and conducts the study and performs all of the laboratory analyses, then it is expected that it would have all of the IP. Issues may arise when the work involves other institutions, or external laboratories (e.g. using their novel equipment or technologies), and all parties must agree the percentage of allocated IP rights and financial income from patents. In other situations, an employee could be the inventor, and there could be an agreement with the employee over IP distribution if using research sponsored by the organisation.

Institutional approval
Many research studies need some kind of local institutional approval before they are conducted, particularly if they involve recruiting participants. This approval will require a review, performed by an independent oversight committee, using the study protocol, PIS, consent form, and any questionnaire (or format of interviews) to be given directly to study participants. The scientific assessment can be quick if there has already been a formal independent review (e.g. regional or national ethics approval), so focus is on the local impact of the study, particularly the use of resources and costs.

Sponsor
The institution acting as the sponsor may have its own internal review of the study design and participant safety and well-being, because it has ultimate responsibility for the study and may have legal responsibility to financially compensate any participants harmed (physically or psychologically) by the

study. The sponsor may be required to ensure that there is sufficient indemnity cover for harm.

Recruiting sites

All institutions from which participants are to be recruited will review the protocol, and any documentation intended for participants. This is because the institution will be partly responsible for conducting the study in accordance with good practice, including ensuring that participants are given informed consent, that adverse events are being recorded and reported (if applicable), and that data are sent to the co-ordinating centre. A site may incur local costs by conducting the study (e.g. additional clinic visits, X-rays or blood tests that are study specific and not part of routine care, and collecting and processing biological samples to be sent to a central biobank) that would not be covered by a grant, so the site will need to agree to meet these costs.

11.3 Conducting the study

After the approvals have been obtained, agreements signed, and potential recruiting sites accepted, the study can proceed. The research team may consider establishing a **Study Master File**, Box 11.7, stored in paper files or electronically. A Study Master File (not all studies need this) ensures that the documents are sufficiently organised, allowing an easy review and audit when required.

Recruiting sites should also keep documents, such as all versions of the protocol; the PIS, signed consent forms; a list of enrolled and screened participants, with their unique identifiers; and any other documents associated with study set-up and conduct, for example, local approval documentation, **site delegation**

Box 11.7 Possible contents of a Study Master File

- Approved study protocol*
- Approved PIS, consent form and any other documents for the subject*
- CRFs*
- Financial aspects of the study (e.g. letter from funder, insurance, and indemnity certificate) and details of participant compensation, if applicable
- All signed agreements between the sponsor and recruiting sites or other parties
- Approval letters and any correspondence from all ethics committees/IRBs
- Approval letter from all recruiting centres
- Curricula vitae of the chief investigator and PI from each site and financial disclosure forms where applicable (to identify any potential conflicts of interest)
- Current laboratory certifications
- List of staff and their responsibilities

*Dated with version numbers.

---

logs (a list of local staff who can work on the study, and their roles), and curriculum vitae of local site staff involved in the study.

Standard Operating Procedures (SOPs)

It is sometimes good practice to have a set of SOPs; particularly for studies that involve recruiting participants. SOPs are summary guidelines, specific to the working practices of the organisation (i.e. the sponsor, co-ordinating centre, or recruiting site). They help to conduct the study to the same standard, and for new staff to quickly familiarise themselves with these practices. SOPs also show that clear and robust systems are in place. Examples of SOPs are:

- Initial site assessment (before recruitment)
- How to set up the sites
- Database development and maintenance
- Database management
- Handling, storing, or posting biological samples
- Recording and reporting adverse events
- Site visits during the study
- Making and reporting protocol amendments
- Statistical considerations (sample size, statistical analysis plan)
- Closing the study (chasing missing data, ensuring that all documentation is stored)

Observational studies based only on data already collected may not require SOPs.

Meetings of study team and investigators

The core study team should meet regularly, particularly during the first few months of the study, and if participants are being recruited. Such meetings could identify and solve problems with recruitment, delivery of questionnaires or interviews, data collection, non-compliance, or issues over study-specific assessments or other key matters.

Investigator meetings are generally held for multicentre studies with at least four or five sites. The lead investigator from each site as well as other key staff should attend. Sites can often learn from the experiences from others. Regular newsletters to everyone involved (at least annually), detailing recruitment and the amount of missing data that needs to be chased up, may be useful.

Monitoring of recruiting sites

Monitoring could include checking that participants really exist, signed consent has been obtained (it required), data have been recorded correctly onto CRFs, and adverse events have been reported. **Source Data Verification (SDV)** is a common method of monitoring performed by pharmaceutical companies for clinical trials, but also in some observational studies. It involves comparing entries on the study-specific CRFs with what is contained in the source data systems, such as medical records. Data could be checked for all participants (100% SDV), or a random proportion of them (e.g. 10% SDV). There is uncertainty whether SDV noticeably changes the main results. Where there are indications that the quality of data from a particular site may be questionable, the research team may decide that it requires some an on-site visit.

Central statistical monitoring [7, 8], using the central electronic study database, can identify errors on key variables, and there are formal statistical methods that can check data for digit preference, compare a variable from one site with the average over all sites to detect outliers, and look for other data anomalies. The site would then be contacted to correct or clarify the anomalies found. Central statistical monitoring is cheaper and easier to perform than full on-site monitoring and SDV.

Monitoring adverse events

Although participants in most observational studies do not suffer any harm, identifying, recording, and reporting **adverse events** may occasionally apply to prospective studies. This could be psychological harm (e.g. due to the nature of the questionnaires or interviews), or physical harm, due to the study-specific assessments.

An adverse event is any untoward or unintended medical occurrence or response, whether it is causally related to the study procedures or not. An adverse event could be the occurrence of a disease or condition that directly affects the participant's health, safety, or well-being, including ability to function. Adverse events are not the same as the disorder of interest. For example, if the study outcome measure is cancer, the occurrence of cancer should not be classified as an adverse event.

Adverse events can be **expected** or **unexpected**, and if expected, they should be listed in the study protocol. An example of an observational study in which some patients may experience adverse events is a translational study, based on obtaining serial tumour samples from lung cancer patients wherever they relapse [4]. Different types of biopsies are used (e.g. endoscopic via the lungs, surgical, and percutaneous core needle biopsy), which depend on the location of the tumour to be sampled (from the lung, or elsewhere). Potential side effects associated with these biopsy procedures include pain, discomfort, bleeding or infection, and so these data should be collected and monitored.

Independent Data Monitoring Committee (IDMC)

This is a group (usually three to five people) of health professionals, a statistician, and other relevant experts with no direct connection to the study. It provides an independent and unbiased review of the study during the recruitment and follow-up periods, and advises the research team. An IDMC is usually only established for prospective cohort studies, especially large multicentre ones, and not required for retrospective studies or those that do not involve contact with participants. The key functions include:

- Identifying poor recruitment and suggesting ways to improve this
- Monitoring the overall conduct of the study, including examining the extent of missing data, particularly for key exposures and outcome measures
- Assessing harm, if applicable

- Examining the collection of biological samples
- Examining data on the main outcome measures and exposures

Before each IDMC meeting, the study statistician and/or co-ordinator prepare a report summarising the main features (as outlined in the bullet points above). After reviewing the report and discussing it with the researchers, the IDMC will either support continuation of the study, or make recommendations to close early. They may also request changes to the study design, protocol, PIS, or consent form, if problems arise or if any of the findings or other evidences indicate this is necessary.

11.4 End of study

Study closure for retrospective studies could be when all the data have been collected and checked. For prospective studies, which involve recruiting participants, closure may be considered in two parts: end of recruitment, and end of follow-up. When the recruitment target has been reached, sites should be informed not to approach further potential participants. This 'closure to recruitment' does not mean the end of the study. The time point at which the study should formally close is usually specified in the protocol, and could be after the last recruited participant has been followed up for the required length of time. The sponsor may need to notify the ethics committee or IRB when accrual and then follow-up has finished. Some studies enter a long-term follow-up phase, collecting key data on exposures and outcomes measures for several more years, as specified in the protocol, so the concept of formal closure may not apply.

The status of the database should be examined, and any missing key information on CRFs from sites should be sought. Some sites fail to submit some data, despite several requests, so the research team could specify how many attempts would be made before accepting the data as missing, with no further chases. When most of this data has been received and entered, the database is downloaded for statistical analysis.

11.5 Regulations

In most countries clinical trials of interventions are associated with clear regulations, but there are fewer regulations for observational studies. Three generally standard regulations aim to ensure that (where applicable):

- There has been independent approval of the research (see page 225).
- Participants have received sufficient information about the study, and provided informed consent (see page 220).
- There is participant anonymity or data confidentiality/protection.

Box 11.8 provides websites that can be used to obtain details about the regulations and guidelines that are used in the UK, US, and elsewhere. Researchers should seek advice from their local institution (e.g. sponsor) if they are unsure. Other regulations exist for storing biological material (in biobanks), sometimes requiring a special licence for laboratories.

Box 11.8 Websites summarising regulations and other guidance for human research studies

UK

1. Health Research Authority (HRA): http://www.hra.nhs.uk
   /http://www.hra.nhs.uk/resources/research-legislation-and-governance/four-nations/2013-2/9/
2. National Research Ethics Service: http://www.nres.nhs.uk/
3. Medical Research Council (MRC): http://www.mrc.ac.uk/PolicyGuidance/EthicsAndGovernance/index.htm

US

1. US Department of Health and Human Services:
   http://www.hhs.gov/ohrp/humansubjects/guidance/45cfr46.html#46.109
2. National Institutes for Health:
   http://grants.nih.gov/grants/policy/hs/index.htm

Summary of guidance from countries internationally
http://www.hhs.gov/ohrp/international/intlcompilation/2014intlcomp.pdf.pdf

---

11.6 Reporting and publishing observational studies

Results of all studies should be reported, usually in a health professional journal, and there are several guidelines on this [9–14]. When reporting observational studies, authors should clarify whether they have only shown association, rather than causation. They should also try to resist the temptation to make their findings appear more 'sensational' than they really are, although journals and the media tend to encourage this through publication bias. Attempting to describe the impact of the results can help address this issue. Importantly, the concept of 'positive' and 'negative' studies should be avoided, because all studies are essentially positive, as they provide useful information about the characteristics of a group of people, and exposures and risk factors; whether practice is changed or not.

The main sections are shown in Box 11.9:

The background section does not have to be long, but should provide a very brief overview of the topic, for example, incidence or prevalence of a disorder, and the key issues associated with it in relation to the paper. There should also be reference to other major work (perhaps focussing on those available at the time the study was developed), and a statement on why the current study was performed.

In the discussion section, it is essential to demonstrate how the findings fit in with other similar studies. If they are discrepant (inconsistent), the authors should attempt to provide an explanation (e.g. the participants might have had different characteristics from those in other studies). The limitations of previous studies could be given, and whether and how the current study

---

Box 11.9   Reporting observational studies: general items to consider (where appropriate)

1. Background and justification
- Summarise the scientific background, and explain why the study was done

2. Methods

2.1 Study type
- Cross-sectional; case-control; retrospective or prospective cohort

2.2 Sampling frame
- Summarise the main characteristics of all sampling frames, including geographical location, and the dates of the first and last participants
- State clearly how participants were identified, or which patient records were used
- Case-control studies: list the matching factors if used

2.3 Participants
- Specify the eligibility criteria for inclusion in the study
- Consider a flow diagram (total number of participants considered, number ineligible with reasons, number drop-outs)
- Patients medical records: state that they were selected consecutively (if not, explain carefully how they were chosen)
- If using an ongoing/closed study, indicate if any participants were excluded for the particular analysis, and why

2.4 Data collection
- Briefly explain how the data were obtained: hospital records (manual or electronic extraction), face-to-face interview, or self-completed questionnaire
- Were data collected directly from the participant, a proxy, or linking to registries?
- Who collected the data and over what time frame?
- Did participants have study-specific assessments (how often, and for how long)?

2.5 Exposures and outcomes
- Define main exposures and outcome measures (including cases and controls); and past or current characteristics
- Briefly explain how they had been measured
- Were standard criteria used to diagnoses the disorder(s) of interest?
- Who assessed the outcomes, and which criteria were used? Were assessors unaware of the exposure status, and was there independent corroboration (e.g. central reviews)?
- If continuous variables were categorised, say how this was done

2.6 Sample size
- Provide details of the sample size, if one was established
- If the study is based on one that already exists, consider a sample size for the specific study objective

2.7 Statistical methods
- Briefly summarise the methods; provide more details if non-standard methods were used
- Explain how missing data were dealt with; consider their effect on the main conclusions

2.8 Biological specimens
- Summarise what type of samples were collected, and how this was done
- Summarise the laboratory methods used to measure biomarkers, e.g. assay type, specialist technical equipment
- Mention whether quality control systems were in place
- Provide details about genotyping methods, and SNPs examined

3. Results

3.1 Participants
- Summary table showing the number of participants, and their main characteristics
- Do this for all participants together, and also according to exposed and unexposed groups (if applicable)
- State the response rate, and say whether or not non-responders are likely to differ from non-responders
- For cohort studies
- What date did follow up (for the purpose of the analysis) end?
- What is the average length of follow up, and total number of person years?
- How many were lost to follow-up (main outcomes were unobtainable)? Did this differ significantly between the exposed and unexposed groups?

3.2 Main results
- Report the number of events if using 'counting people' or time-to-event outcome measures; for 'taking measurements on people' report the standard deviations
- Summarise the amount of missing data for the key analyses
- Show at least one figure (diagram) of the main findings
- Provide both unadjusted and adjusted effect sizes (if applicable), and state which confounding factors were allowed for
- Describe the association (e.g. small, moderate, or large), and whether clinically important
- Provide 95% CIs and p-values for the main results
- Could major bias or confounding distort the main findings?
- Provide any subgroup analyses, and briefly explain why these are reported

4. Discussion and conclusions

4.1 The study
- Provide a brief overview of the most important findings
- Provide some key strengths and limitations (of the design/analysis)

4.2 Supporting evidence
- Always provide evidence from other (ideally independent and large) studies, including those that are inconsistent with the study results, and on biological plausibility

4.3 What next?
- Are the conclusions on associations or risk factors sufficiently strong?
- If making conclusions about causality, discuss the features (Boxes 2.7 & 6.9)
- Discuss generalisability, and whether or not the findings could apply elsewhere
- Explain the clinical importance and implications of the findings (e.g. prevention, diagnosis/detection, or treatment)
- Is it appropriate to recommend changing practice, to confirm existing practice, or recommend further research (and outline key design)?

Based on some items from reference 6.

overcomes these. Finally, the researchers should always summarise the contribution their study and the results has made to clinical practice or knowledge, which may also be influenced by other studies.

Most journals restrict the number of words, tables, and figures, so researchers must present their study (which may have taken several years to conduct) concisely. This can be partly achieved by presenting numerical results in tables or figures, rather than in the text. Many journals are now available electronically via the internet, allowing supplementary text, tables, and figures that do not appear in the printed version to be provided in an online appendix. The contents of the appendix are not included in the word or table/figure count. Including an appendix allows researchers to provide all the necessary details about their study and the results, making it more likely that journal editors and external reviewers will review the paper favourably, because they are able to assess the paper properly.

There is increasing interest in providing a simple (lay) summary of the main findings to study participants, particularly for prospective cohort studies. This could be provided via a website.

Conflict of interests
Many publishers require a declaration of financial support received for a study, any relevant patents, and any connection with the manufacturers of products or devices used. Conflict of interests, sometimes referred to as competing interests, arises when the professional judgement concerning the validity and interpretation of research could be influenced by financial gain, or professional advantage or rivalry. Authors should state who funded the study, because this may have influenced their interpretation of the data (e.g. indicating that the results are more generalisable than they really are), perhaps subconsciously. Authors should also declare any personal financial interests associated with the paper, such as fees they may have received from suppliers of laboratory materials or equipment associated with translational research, in order to allow the reader to judge whether this may have affected the study conduct and interpretation of the results.

11.7 Key points
- Most observational studies must go through several stages from developing the concept to publication of the findings.
- Sufficient resources must be secured in order to conduct and complete the study in a timely fashion.
- Having a clearly written and concise protocol helps the research team and other centres (sites) involved in recruiting participants or collecting data.
- Informed consent, anonymity, and data confidentiality are key issues that need to be clarified for a particular study, and researchers should be aware of any guidelines and regulations on these. There may also be regulations on the creation and maintenance of a biobank.
- Study-specific CRFs and a good electronic database are important for collecting and storing data.

- Agreements or contracts may be needed between institutions involved in conducting a study, and conditions for IP should be clarified.
- All studies should be published, regardless of the findings, and the content of the report should contain necessary details for a proper review by readers.

References

1. Hackshaw AK. How to Write a Grant Application: For Health Professionals and Life Sciences Researchers. Wiley-Blackwell. First Edition (2011).
2. Kho ME, Duffett M, Willison DJ, Cook DJ, Brouwers MC. Written informed consent and selection bias in observational studies using medical records: systematic review. BMJ 2009;338:b866. doi:10.1136/bmj.b866.
3. Bookman EB, Langehorne AA, Eckfeldt JH, Glass KC, Jarvik GP, Klag M, et al.; NHLBI Working Group. Reporting genetic results in research studies: summary and recommendations of an NHLBI working group. Am J Med Genet A 2006;140(10):1033–40.
4. TRAcking Non-small Cell Lung Cancer Evolution Through Therapy (Rx) (TRACERx). http://clinicaltrials.gov/show/NCT01888601.
5. Epi Info, Version 7. US Centers for Disease Control and Prevention. http://wwwn.cdc.gov/epiinfo/7/. Accessed 20 May 2014.
6. Statistical analysis in social science (SPSS). http://www-01.ibm.com/software/analytics/spss/. Accessed 20 May 2014.
7. Kirkwood A, Cox T, Hackshaw A. Application of methods for central statistical monitoring in clinical trials. Clin Trials 2013;10:783–806.
8. Baigent C, Harrell FE, Buyse M, Emberson JR, Altman DG. Ensuring trial validity by data quality assurance and diversification of monitoring methods. Clin Trials 2008;5:49–55.
9. von Elm E, Altman DG, Egger M, Pocock SJ, Gøtzsche PC, Vandenbroucke JP; STROBE Initiative. The Strengthening the Reporting of Observational Studies in Epidemiology (STROBE) statement: guidelines for reporting observational studies. J Clin Epidemiol 2008;61(4):344–9.
10. Riley RD, Abrams KR, Sutton AJ, Lambert PC, Jones DR, Heney D, Burchill SA. Reporting of prognostic markers: current problems and development of guidelines for evidence-based practice in the future. Br J Cancer 2003;88(8):1191–8.
11. Bossuyt PM, Reitsma JB, Bruns DE, Gatsonis CA, Glasziou PP, Irwig LM, et al.; Standards for Reporting of Diagnostic Accuracy. Towards complete and accurate reporting of studies of diagnostic accuracy: the STARD initiative. Clin Radiol 2003;58(8):575–80.
12. McShane LM, Altman DG, Sauerbrei W, Taube SE, Gion M, Clark GM; Statistics Subcommittee of the NCI-EORTC Working Group on Cancer Diagnostics. Reporting recommendations for tumor marker prognostic studies. J Clin Oncol 2005;23(36):9067–72.
13. Little J, Higgins JP, Ioannidis JP, Moher D, Gagnon F, von Elm E, et al.; STrengthening the REporting of Genetic Association Studies. STrengthening the REporting of Genetic Association Studies (STREGA): an extension of the STROBE statement. PLoS Med 2009; 6(2):e22. doi:10.1371/journal.pmed.1000022.
14. Altman DG, McShane LM, Sauerbrei W, Taube SE. Reporting Recommendations for Tumor Marker Prognostic Studies (REMARK): explanation and elaboration. PLoS Med 2012;9(5):e1001216. doi:10.1371/journal.pmed.1001216.

Index

A Concise Guide to Observational Studies in Healthcare, First Edition. Allan Hackshaw.
© 2015 John Wiley & Sons, Ltd. Published 2015 by John Wiley & Sons, Ltd.